W9-AAX-524

The
Well Path

The Well Path

Lose 20 Pounds,
Reverse the Aging Process,
Change Your Life

JAMÉ HESKETT, M.D.

HARPER WAVE

This book contains advice and information relating to health care. It is not intended to replace medical advice and should be used to supplement rather than replace regular care by your doctor. It is recommended that you seek your physician's advice before embarking on any medical program or treatment. All efforts have been made to assure the accuracy of the information contained in this book as of the date of publication. The publisher and the author disclaim liability for any medical outcomes that may occur as a result of applying the methods suggested in this book.

FIRST EDITION

Designed by Kris Tobiassen / Matchbook Digital

Library of Congress Cataloging-in-Publication Data has been applied for.

ISBN: 978-0-06-241553-0

16 17 18 19 20   OV/RRD   10 9 8 7 6 5 4 3 2 1

This book is dedicated to
Sue and Bill Dalton,
for believing that I could do something special
with a little place called WellPath.

A woman is the full circle. Within her is the power to create, to nurture, to transform.

—DIANE MARIECHILD

Contents

PART FOUR: Start Souping

The Well Path

Introduction

I see naked people.

Lots of naked people. As a doctor, I see unclothed females of all ages, sizes, and shapes every day. Ninety-nine percent of them arrive at my office stressed out, frustrated, and exhausted. They tell me they've been trying everything under the sun to lose unwanted pounds and look younger, with no success.

Before the naked part of a consultation, I sit down with new patients to have a talk in my office. "How can I help you?" I ask.

Often, tears well in their eyes. I think it's an automatic reaction to the shame of feeling like a failure because the number on the scale or their appearance doesn't reflect the goals they've set for themselves. These are extremely high-functioning women. They are successful New York City career ladies and great moms with impeccable style, but this one simple thing completely undoes them. They are women who have the other areas of their lives "together," but they can't get a handle on their health. They try to hide their vulnerability, but as we talk it becomes difficult.

I encourage them to let it out. These women are already stretched beyond their breaking point. I've heard variations of "I've been dieting my whole life and can't lose weight" and "I work out like a fiend and still have cellulite" every day of my career. They've received the same message from every source available to them: To lose weight, you have to eat less and exercise more. They work so hard to follow this advice with so much good intention and determination that I wish I could give them gold medals. In every other aspect of life, they succeed. But in this particular area, according to their own impossibly high standards, they fail and then they blame themselves.

The stakes are high. These women are fighting for their health and quality of life, for their ability to do their life's work, to be good role models for their children, and to be happy. They're trying to free themselves from the burden of excess weight, to slow down the aging process, and to decrease their odds of developing the diseases and conditions associated with being overweight and aging.

What they don't yet realize is that "trying everything" is precisely *why* "nothing works."

Let's define *everything*:

Chronic dieting and calorie restriction

Trying every new fad diet or exercise regimen, even if it doesn't feel good

Taking questionable supplements to shed pounds

Juice cleansing or detoxing on a regular basis

Exercising to exhaustion or injury or, the flip side, not working out hard enough to break a sweat

Living with the stress, anxiety, and depression of feeling like a failure

The emotional and physical toll of this struggle is enormous. With each new diet or exercise class, women start out with high expectations and wind up disappointed, frustrated, guilt-ridden, and ashamed when they don't get the results they want or when the results are not sustainable. One trip on this emotional roller coaster would be hard enough, but most of the women I meet have been on this ride for years, even decades.

But the toll isn't only emotional; it's also biological. Women unknowingly dismantle their healthy bodily functions—including their metabolism—by dieting and overexercising. In their attempt to "try everything" they undermine the delicate balance of their hormones—the body's chemical messengers that are involved in regulating everything from weight to skin elasticity to energy levels. In their quest to be strong, vibrant, and healthy, women who "try everything" create a weak and sick internal environment. Their bodies are eventually thrown so off-kilter that positive changes become next to impossible to make. All of their dutiful hours logged on the treadmill are a perfect metaphor for their efforts: They have truly been running in place, going nowhere fast.

As they get older, the panic volume goes up. "Losing weight in my twenties was so simple," women often say. "But now, I'm stuck." When they were younger, it was easier to lose weight for many reasons, but one was that their bodies weren't broken down yet by decades of inconsistent nutrition and exercise. The unfortunate irony is that the longer and harder they've been trying to lose weight, the more difficult it is for them to succeed. "I'm a mess, and I don't want to feel this way," they tell me. "You're my last hope. I saw you use that fat-zapping laser machine on *Dr. Oz*, and I want to give it a try."

I understand their desire for a "cure." I have become well known for demonstrating aesthetic machines on TV, so new patients often hope these high-tech tools are the miracle solution to their weight-loss woes. But that's not how long-term weight loss works.

Technology can be a powerful tool, but it won't solve the problem of an imbalanced body or a yo-yo lifestyle. Treatments require a commitment of time and money, and they alone cannot solve the underlying issues that are causing weight gain or aging in the first place. As a first step, I suggest to my patients that they try my holistic strategies. They'll invest less time, get better results, and change the trajectory of their health and longevity. And the cost? Next to nothing.

They'll also bond with other women, gain tons of energy, eat fabulously, sleep like a dream, cure a host of bothersome problems, and feel empowered by their proactivity. All without feeling deprived. They will achieve homeostasis—a state of optimal health where your whole body is in balance, humming along, every system working in perfect harmony with one another—as well as lose fat and slow the aging process from the inside out.

Nine out of ten women say, "I've *tried* every program out there already. I don't even know what homeostasis means." In their desperation, they just want something that works fast. My approach to wellness, they wrongly suspect, will be just another empty promise.

The Well Path, as I call it, is not a diet. I don't believe in elimination or restrictive diets. I don't even like to say (or type) the word *diet*. It's been my personal and professional experience that when a woman says or thinks the D-word, she will gain five pounds by the end of the week.

So if it's not a diet, what is it? The Well Path is a series of small steps that, cumulatively, move your body back into balance and allow you to thrive. Part of the Path does involve eating—but not eliminating. I believe in *adding* nutrients to food you like, not taking things away. "Nutrify" is a much better word than "diet." The Well Path gives you the tools you need to rebuild and strengthen your body and mind. The goal isn't starvation, it's homeostasis. Fat melts away and is replaced with healthy muscle. Energy soars. Depression and stress levels drop. Skin glows. Cells renew and regenerate faster than they die off, literally turning back the clock on aging.

Restrictive eaters are *not* in homeostasis.

Neither are compulsive exercisers, couch potatoes, insomniacs, or workaholics.

Signs that you're not in homeostasis include the inability to sleep or poor-quality sleep; constipation; loose bowels; bloating; cravings for caffeine and sweet, salty, and starchy foods; late-night binge eating; excess abdominal fat; cellulite; dull skin tone; feeling stressed out, overwhelmed, and exhausted; and being forgetful or having a sense that you are not as sharp as you used to be. When you're not in homeostasis, you're basically on life support. Your body is in a chronic reactive, defensive state and is just doing what it needs to survive. It can't, and won't, thrive in constant crisis. My strategies are designed to change the body's internal environment from "stop" to "go," from sick to healthy, fat to lean, tired to energized.

Signs that you *are* in homeostasis are good-quality sleep; easily falling and staying asleep; healthy daily bowel movements; no sugar or caffeine cravings; normal hunger pangs; decreasing abdominal fat; smooth and glowing skin; energy to spare; well-managed stress; healthy libido; and sharper mental function, including improved memory.

Along with my diet- and fitness-obsessed patients, I see just as many women who are lost in the ocean of conflicting information out there about health, aging, and weight. They don't know where to start a wellness plan, so they let it slide for years, gaining weight and losing their health in their inertia. No matter what shape my patients are in when they first set foot on the Well Path, they can typically expect to achieve homeostasis in about a month. Women who were on multiple medications and couldn't walk up a flight of stairs have been able to minimize their pills and hike up a mountain.

You can't get results like that with just a laser.

Any path to success in life and in health has to start with a strong desire to make real, lasting, positive changes. When you incorporate my sustainable, simple changes into your life, real change is possible. We're going to take it one step at a time, one meal at a time, one day at a time. It is as simple, and effective, as that.

My Story

Finding and stepping along a healthy path is how I live my life. I walk the walk, big-time. But it wasn't always that way.

When I look back at my life, I see it as a progression of taking one step at a time to reach where I am now. I grew up in Los Angeles. Although I have blond hair, I was far from a California Girl proto-type—I was always on the chubby side. I'm pretty sure hot dogs and bologna were major staples of my childhood. From elementary school on, weight was a constant battle for me, and I remember the first crush I ever had told me that I was too fat for him to like me. The pain of that comment is still familiar even thirty-three years later. I had other struggles, too. Although I had parents who loved and supported me, I always felt like I didn't fit in because I wasn't pretty, thin, smart, or talented enough. My parents didn't have a lot of financial resources, so I worked my own way through college and medical school doing phone sales and waitressing, eventually becoming a doctor specializing in family health.

My life goal had always been to help women reach their full potential. Overcoming obstacles had (has) been the struggle of my own life, and if I could help others with theirs, that would be my definition of success. I joined a medical practice and started working with women and children, often advising them how to lose excess weight. I can count on two hands what I learned about nutrition in medical school, but I stuck with the standard message: Eat less, exercise more. Four words that have doomed countless weight-loss efforts over the past few decades.

Well, it didn't work for my patients or for me. Again and again, I saw the proof in practice: Diets were stressful and depressing and caused my patients to gain more weight over time. I knew that if my patients could free themselves of the obsessive distraction of diet plans and the emotional devastation of chronic failure, they'd be happier, healthier, and more successful in every aspect of their lives. I started to develop sustainable, successful strategies for weight loss and wellness and test them out with my patients—this was the foundation for the Well Path.

During this period of my life, I was living in Seattle. I had married and had my daughter, Olivia. Professionally, I was thriving and in the midst of developing a wellness center for women. But on the eve of signing a long-term lease for my future business, I stopped and took stock. It had always been a dream of mine to live and work in New York City. If I signed that Seattle lease, there was no turning back. The very next day, I found a real estate ad in a wrongly delivered *New York Times* that read, "Day spa for sale, Upper East Side." I flew across the country and walked sixty blocks up Madison Avenue on a beautiful spring day to find a dump. A dump with potential.

One look was enough. I had found my new wellness center. A generous friend lent me the money to buy it. Six weeks later, in May 2001, I moved to New York City with my husband and my eighteen-month-old daughter. I established my practice and had another child, Sam. It seemed great on paper: two kids, Upper East Side medical practice, happily married. But our marriage was not a happy one, and eventually we separated. A bitter, ugly divorce and custody battle followed. I poured my heart into my children and my soul into my work, and eventually gave up, peacefully, on finding another mate after a few years of dating disappointments.

And then I met the man who'd change my mind about getting married again.

Dave is ten years my junior and an amazing stepfather. We decided to have a child together, and I got pregnant with Cole at forty-two after two miscarriages and a tubal pregnancy. Not only was my body a mess from all the hormonal ups and downs, I was considered a high-risk pregnancy and my doctor advised me to take it easy. For nine months I barely moved and ate way too much. My son Cole should have been named Ben or Jerry! My net gain from that pregnancy was sixty pounds.

I lost almost no weight after Cole was born, I was out of shape, and I felt powerless against the pounds on the scale. Every time I tried to imagine what it would take to get rid of the weight, I thought, "There's just no way." Despite having coached many patients in my same position, it still felt like an overwhelming challenge. Until that moment, I hadn't really known what it was like to be at the bottom of a weight-loss mountain and not being able to see the top.

I would have to apply my methods to my own situation, including the strategy of keeping my head down and watching my feet take one step at a time.

Every time I caught myself looking for the endpoint and feeling overwhelmed, I reminded myself that I didn't have to lose sixty pounds today. I only had to have a nice lunch, take a walk later, spend time with friends and family, and enjoy life. I didn't panic. I stayed on the path and I kept moving forward. Six months later, I had lost it all and was fit and full of vitality.

When I look back at what it took to get there, I am amazed at how simple it was. The series of small steps started out with one meal. Then it was one exercise class. Then it was a whole day, a whole week, whatever I could handle doing. If I tried something drastic and unsustainable, I could feel myself wanting to quit. So I took a deep breath and refocused on taking one step, one meal, one class, to get back on the path to the top of the mountain. Anything can be achieved when you break it up into small, manageable components that can be sustained and integrated into your daily life.

This personal experience helped me further hone the Well Path. I know for a fact that losing twenty or more pounds is a matter of keeping your head down and taking small steps, one at a time. Climb your hill (not someone else's) doing things you like, and you'll arrive at homeostasis with a smile of pride on your face. Take rests. Soak up the sun. Smell the flowers. Bring other people along as you go. Losing weight and reversing the aging process can be *fun*. People laugh at me when I say this, but only at first. After they've been on the Path for a while, they laugh with knowing relief, not skepticism.

No matter where you are on your journey right now, you are capable of greatness. No matter what shape you're in, you can return to the natural state of optimal functioning you were intrinsically designed for. You can work with your body instead of against it. Perpetually cycling between expectation and disappointment distracts women from reaching higher goals and from succeeding at their life's work, whatever that might be.

My higher goal, my life's work, is to help women prioritize their health and well-being so they can achieve *their* higher goals and succeed at *their* life's work. Nothing can stop a woman who is healthy, energized, and confident. Everyone benefits when you feel good: the kids, your partner, your colleagues and community. In my twenty-four years of practicing both traditional and alternative medicine, I have guided hundreds of women along this clear, brightly lit Path to wellness. Before you read any of my specific directions, know that the only thing you have to cut out of your life is fear of failing. No more insane dieting, cleansing, suffering, and churning away on an elliptical to nowhere. That dark period of your life is over. Time now to heal from the inside out, feel better, look *amazing*, live longer, and finally get rid of the extra weight.

PART ONE

The Truth about Weight Loss and Aging

1.

What Prevents Change

The very first, biggest step on the Well Path is making the decision to change. It's not easy to put aside the habits you've become used to and to reframe the way you think about health and weight loss. So before we get you started on a new path, I want to take a moment to help you understand why your previous path isn't working. Most of us have accepted certain beliefs about our health—the headlines you see plastered on magazines and websites that influence the choices you make at the grocery store, in the kitchen, at the gym, at work. But many of these messages are misunderstood or simply false. Instead of helping you lose weight and increase vitality, they turn out to be change blockers. So let's start with a little myth busting.

Change Blocker #1: Dieting Is Healthy

Many of my patients have been D-wording since they were teenagers and have never experienced how amazing it feels to have a balanced body in homeostasis. Their eating has been disordered—chronic deprivation *is* an eating disorder—since adolescence. They are stuck in a pattern of behavior that is so ingrained they don't feel right unless they're dieting, even though dieting makes them unhappy. Which means: They don't feel right unless they're unhappy.

Many of my patients diet out of habit. They're not doing it because it works—if it did, they wouldn't need to diet for years on end. A lot of the women I see in my practice follow an eating plan because without it they would feel untethered. They want the structure. They feel better when someone else tells them what they can and can't eat, when their eating is tightly controlled by rules. Nothing gives them more anxiety than feeling out of control. On the surface, diets seem to offer control. But when they fail—usually in a no-holds-barred binge—these women feel more out of control than ever. Soon they're consumed with shame and guilt over their "failure" and start looking for a new system to help them control themselves.

I appreciate that having a course of action can be motivating. On the Well Path, you will be on course. But the action you'll take is NOT restricting food. It's taking positive, self-loving steps that will gradually shift your appetite so that you begin to crave nutrient-dense food. It's not that you aren't "allowed" to have less healthy foods. You can have them. But you won't want them.

Five Types of Eaters

Everyone has their own habits when it comes to food, but I've found over the years that many of my patients tend to fit into one of the five categories below. Each eating "type" is also clearly aligned with certain psychological and emotional types. Which type are you?

The Food Eliminator. Anyone who follows rules like "no carbs/no fat/no gluten/no white food/no solid food/no fruit/nothing cavemen didn't eat." Elimination is always appealing to dieters because it gives them a simple regimen, a food or food group to draw an X over. The problem is, cutting out any food group is not optimal from a nutritional standpoint. We need it all—carbs, fat, protein, fiber, fruit—to stay healthy, lose fat, and grow muscle. If you eat 5,000 calories of protein, for example, you will still feel hungry because your body *is* hungry for other nutrients. Also, if you are left with options that are unsatisfying or get boring fast, it makes the forbidden fruit all the more tempting.

The Out-of-the-Box Eater. Now that so-called healthy, low-calorie food is widely available in packaged form, some women rely on frozen or prepared meals for the bulk of their calories. This type of eating is the main culprit of late-night bingeing. Your body demands nutrients. If you haven't supplied them throughout the day because all you've been eating is packaged cereal bars or frozen low-fat lasagna, your brain will override your willpower and force you to eat until your body gets what it wants.

The Meal Skipper. Too busy to eat. Not hungry in the morning. Too tired to cook dinner. The Meal Skipper might eat healthfully, but the erratic timing of her meals causes her metabolism to slow down. If your body doesn't get food regularly, it will, by default, go into starvation mode and hold on to energy stores for dear life.

The Overeater. Many of my patients fall into this category. They know what's good for them, including healthy fats, home cooking, and keeping a regular eating schedule. They just eat too much of the good stuff. It's about quality *and* quantity. They bake ten flour-free cookies and eat all of them. Or they drizzle tons of olive oil on a salad or smother it with chopped nuts.

The Diet Cycler. These women leap from one restrictive plan to the next. They are always on a diet or planning the next one. Most of the diets deprive the body of food groups and/or nutrients and disrupt the metabolism and endocrine function. Their bodies never get the chance to recover before they're on to the next plan. The logistical nightmare of trying to remember the rules of whatever plan they're on is so consuming that the diet cycler's life shrinks down to the size of a single plate. After she rebels against her self-imposed rules, she blames herself for failing instead of blaming the true culprit—the diet itself.

Do you recognize yourself in one or more of these eating types? If so, you're not alone. The first step is to be aware of your particular style, and keep an eye out when bad tendencies sneak up on you. The only healthy "type" of eater is someone who is mindful about her choices, responds to the messages her body is sending, eats when hungry and stops when full, and enjoys every bite. Within weeks on the Well Path, my patients' eating habits are transformed. The elimination and obsession and unhealthy habits are replaced with genuine curiosity about nutrition and a love for food that feeds their cells and fuels their metabolism.

Change Blocker #2: Magic Bullets Are Real

Hope is more powerful than failure. For this reason, it's easy to sell a miracle pill or product to desperate people. You intuitively know that no ingredient exists that will make weight drop off your body effortlessly without changing your eating habits or lifestyle. The quick fix dream won't die because it's a compelling fantasy. Who wouldn't want to drop ten pounds overnight?

A supplement or ingredient won't make you confident, thin, or strong. But restoring your health, one step at a time, will change your body and mind so profoundly it will *feel* like magic. The magic bullet doesn't exist.

Change Blocker #3: If You Lost Ten Pounds, Then You'd Be Happy

The number on the scale doesn't mean anything. It doesn't tell you how fit you are, how much muscle you have, how energetic you are, or how well you've gotten through the day without going nuts. I often ask patients, "When you get to that dream number, how will your life change exactly?" Will they have a new apartment? A new husband? Better kids? A better job? Smaller bills? Usually, they don't even know the answer. They have an amorphous idea about having more confidence and feeling better about themselves if they hit their goal.

I ask, "Would you feel confident and better about yourself if you ate well every day and were stronger and happier?"

They nod, of course. Happiness and health are not measured in pounds, inches, or sizes. The benefits of good health and wellness are comprehensive and multidimensional. On a diet, there is only one measure of success—a smaller number—that doesn't take your overall wellness into account. On the Well Path, there are many ways to succeed.

Change Blocker #4: Losing Weight Has to Hurt

The conventional wisdom is that in order to lose weight and get in shape, you have to suffer. No pain no gain, right?

Wrong. Change is sustainable only if you enjoy making it. Most women are so caught up in the struggle to lose weight—keeping their eyes focused on the prize—that they pride themselves on their ability to overcome discomfort. If you asked them, "Is your diet joyful?" they'd laugh until they cried into their fat-free yogurt. As humans, we're hardwired to shut down metabolically during deprivation and to rebel against pain. When our bodies can't take deprivation and pain anymore, we go *hard* in the other direction and eat to excess. We're also hardwired to replenish lost stores of energy (meaning fat) after depleting them. But when we move and are fueled properly *and consistently*, our bodies become metabolically efficient, making weight loss a pleasure.

Change Blocker #5: Weight Loss Is Mind over Matter

Despite the number of books, TV shows, and articles that suggest otherwise, you can't override your body's needs. Instead of trying to be the boss of your body and telling it what to do, here's a radical idea:

Listen to it. Your body is constantly trying to communicate with you. Sometimes it might say, "That's enough sitting for today. You need to move and get some fresh air." Other times it might subtly suggest that you drink some water or go to bed early. These messages aren't always communicated in obvious ways—like when you're ravenously hungry. The clues might be subtle, such as a craving for a certain food to signal a vitamin deficiency, a slight change in skin color, or a minor cramp or dull pain.

The great tragedy of being on a diet, pushing yourself beyond your limits with exercise, or mindlessly eating unhealthy food is losing touch with that internal sensitivity to what your body actually needs. The rare patient takes the time to be quiet and listen to her body. Most ignore their body's signal for nutrition, work out past their limits, and overconsume empty calories. Exhausted and out of balance, they react by drinking too much coffee, grabbing a candy bar for a quick source of energy, or purge out of guilt.

On the Well Path, you will stop ignoring and start listening. Your body knows better than you what it needs for optimal functioning. Stop needing to be in charge. That won't help you reach homeostasis. All of the stress, control, disappointment, shame, and guilt are what got you here. Having fun, eating well, and listening to your body will get you where you want to go.

Change Blocker #6: Failure Is All Your Fault

Dieting makes you gain weight. Excessive exercise makes you weak. Overeating makes you fat. The impact of chronic stress, starvation, and bingeing over the years will eventually ruin your ability to lose weight and accelerate the aging process. It's heartbreaking to see how hard women work to no avail. And then they blame themselves.

Self-abusing thoughts like "I eat like a pig" and "I have no discipline" only make matters worse. You are not a failure for rebelling against a diet. The nature of your body is to seek out food when it gets even a whiff of deprivation, real or imagined. You are not to blame for eating a piece of cake. Cake is just cake. It's not a recrimination of your entire life.

I advise my patients to stop setting themselves up for failure. Their destructive habits are "outside in" thinking. It's the messed-up belief that if you're thin, you're somehow more valuable. "Inside out" thinking means your outside will shine radiantly when you're healthy on the inside.

Our bodies should function exquisitely. We were designed to be in balance and to chug along like a well-oiled machine. But we've altered our physiology by adapting to myths that are constructed for profit and sold to us at a dear price. Dieting misconceptions—the rules many women live by—are actually Change Blockers that, long-term, are detrimental to your health and to your weight.

Manipulating your nature is not the way to thrive.

The eat less/exercise more model slows fat metabolism, accelerates aging, and causes hormonal imbalance. I'll explain the science of that in the next three chapters.

The Only "Do" and "Don't" You'll Ever Need

I get so annoyed when I scroll through my Facebook newsfeed and see a dozen articles from various magazines and blogs with titles like "Ten Exercises to Get a Bikini Butt." I'm just like everyone else. I think, *I'd like a bikini butt*, whatever that is, and I click through. The suggestions are nothing new, but in my head I add them to the list of things to try. I see another list, for "Eight Tricks for a Flat Belly." At the end of the day, I've got 200 new things to do. I get so much anxiety reading these articles, like I've got to learn it all and do it all. I've tagged a bunch of them (because I feel the pressure to do them), and guess what? I have never done any of them.

I have my own list of Don'ts and Dos for you to "like":

The only Don't you'll ever need: Don't feel pressured to read and execute the advice in those articles. Doing the eight or ten or twenty tricks and tips to improve an isolated muscle group is trees-not-forest thinking. Your health is bigger than your butt (no matter how big it might be). Just doing squats and kickbacks won't rebalance hormones, stoke cellular repair, or wake up a sleepy metabolism.

The only Do you'll ever need: Do go outside and play. To access the forest of your health, take a long walk in the forest, or wherever you prefer, with a close friend. Spending a pleasant afternoon in nature with people or alone at peace will trigger a multitude of positive physiological changes that improve your health holistically. And if a few mountains lure you to climb them, you might just notice some changes in your tush.

2.

The Truth about Metabolism

If you've ever tried to lose weight, I know you're familiar with the word "metabolism"—at least as it pertains to weight loss. You may have been told that having a fast metabolism is a good thing, and having a slow metabolism is a bad thing. You may have been told that the best thing you can do to lose weight is to "boost" your metabolism. But what is metabolism, exactly?

In order to stay alive, your body must maintain a number of metabolic functions—that is, bodily functions that require energy from your cells. We metabolize while walking down the street, thinking, breathing, digesting. Pretty much everything we do, from blinking your eyes to running a marathon, requires energy. A "fast metabolism," as it's colloquially known, means your body easily converts stored fat to energy for all of your body's needs. A "slow metabolism" means your body is stingy about giving up fat for fuel.

Fat cells aren't like skin or liver cells. They're uniquely plastic, expanding, leaking, and changing in your body all the time. When our body's most common fat molecules, triglycerides, leak out of fat cell membranes, they are "free," able to travel in the bloodstream to your cells and the liver to be metabolized for energy. The process of coaxing triglycerides, aka free fatty acids (FFAs), out of those cells is complex. Hormones, enzymes, and other chemical messengers are needed to unlock the fat cells. The basic metabolic pathway for fat goes something like this:

Hormones and enzymes signal to your fat cells to leak FFAs.

The FFAs are absorbed into your blood vessels, which are threaded through the spaces in your body between cells.

Your flowing blood carries the FFAs to the liver, your body's filtration system.

More hormones and enzymes do the job of figuring out where the freshly filtered FFAs need to go.

The FFAs are then sent to your muscles, brain, and all the other organs that require energy at any given moment. The FFAs are consumed as fuel, much like your car consumes gas to make the wheels go around.

To streamline this process, your body needs balanced hormones and enzymes, a robust circulatory system, a clean liver, and well-hydrated muscles and organs with well-oxygenated and nutrient-fed cells. If you are out of balance hormonally or nutritionally, your fat cells are reluctant to give up FFAs, and your metabolism slows to a crawl. From an evolutionary standpoint, it makes sense—our bodies depend on this well-orchestrated storage and release of fat for survival in times of scarcity.

When your bodily systems are in balance, your metabolism is enabled to move more quickly—this is the "fast metabolism" everyone speaks of with such awe and reverence. A healthy metabolism is the result of a healthy body. You can convert fat to fuel easily when your body is healthy enough to quickly release FFAs and transport it to where it's needed most.

Your metabolism is one of the most amazing, dynamic, and important systems in your body. You can't live without it. Improper nutrition, erratic exercise, inadequate rest, and stress compromise this vital system by disrupting hormones and enzymes, clogging circulation, bogging down the liver with toxins, dehydrating muscles, and deoxygenating and starving organ cells.

In other words: Dieting breaks down your metabolism.

How Dieting Slows Metabolism

Your body doesn't care how you look in a pair of jeans. It was designed to keep you from starving to death during a famine. In response to caloric deprivation, your brain receives a flood of hormonal signals that increases cravings, hunger, and appetite, prompting you to eat whatever is immediately available and to store fat even if you've already got plenty to spare. In fact, humans don't have a regulatory system that signals "okay, you're fat enough now." Adipocytes (fat cells) will expand and multiply unchecked. Our capacity to store fat is limited only by death—and if you get big enough, your body will kill you.

Dieting works against nature by enlisting your body's "Must eat! Must store fat!" survival mechanism. Even thinking about dieting can have this effect. The brain immediately becomes aware of the impending deprivation and will respond to protect you, a response you cannot overcome with willpower. According to a March 2015 article in the journal *Appetite*, researchers found that self-deprivation of any type led to increased eating. The eighty-five subjects were shown a funny movie. One group was told not to laugh or react to it. The other group could react naturally. After being psychologically "primed"—a sneaky method of subconsciously leading someone to think about an idea or behavior—via a word puzzle with words like "diet" and "weight," the two groups were offered snacks. The first group ate significantly more than the second group. Their restriction wasn't even about food, and yet it was so depleting on a subconscious level, they ate more without having any idea why or that it was happening. So tell yourself "No more cookies!" or "Don't get angry at my boss today," and watch what happens.

The old wisdom used to be that restricting overall calories would make you skinny. The less you ate, the skinnier you'd be. It's certainly true that if you were starved in a prison, say, with no access to a wide variety of food, you would lose weight. Your muscles and fat would waste away, and your metabolic rate would drop in order to keep you alive. If you were then released from prison and started to eat normally again, your intake of calories would exceed your crawling metabolic rate. As a result, the pounds would pile on *rapidly*.

I've seen this phenomenon occur in women with eating disorders. One woman I worked with had starved herself down from 140 to 100 pounds over the course of four months. With therapy and the support of her family, she was able to start eating normally again—and gained *eighty* pounds in three months. In the span of only eight months, she lost forty pounds, and gained eighty.

I wish I could say this is an extreme example. But how many of us have dieted to lose ten pounds and then gained back twenty? I've observed in my practice that for every one pound you lose on a month-long diet, you can expect to put on two within a month of the diet's completion.

I came across a fascinating study recently in the journal *Family Practice*. Researchers at the State University of New York at Stony Brook put their subjects—twenty women from fifty-six to seventy years old—on a diet of 1,100 calories per day for eleven weeks. Researchers monitored the subjects' food intake to make sure they adhered to the plan. When the eleven weeks were over, the women were measured and weighed.

On such paltry rations, it's no wonder the women lost weight. On average, they lost 9 percent of their total weight, 5 percent of their lean muscle mass, and 15 percent of their body fat. Their resting metabolic rate also decreased by *15 percent*, meaning their ability to convert fat to energy slowed down significantly, nearly double the percentage of the weight they lost. What's more, their metabolic rate didn't pick up speed when the diet ended, predicting that they'd regain all the weight they lost and then some.

Your resting metabolic rate slows down on a very low calorie diet (VLCD). Most researchers and medical experts consider an intake of less than 1,200 per day in the VLCD range. Why does eating less than

1,200 calories per day impact your metabolism in this way? Here are a few reasons:

Loss of lean muscle mass. If you aren't eating adequate carbs and protein, your body can't generate new muscle or maintain the muscle mass you already have. In fact, without an adequate supply of dietary amino acids (which are found in protein), your body will consume your existing muscles for its basic energy requirements. It's like eating yourself from the inside out. On a very low calorie diet (VLCD), you literally make yourself weaker by losing muscle.

A sedentary lifestyle. Not many people on a VLCD are doing much of anything besides dragging themselves through the day. With so few calories coming in and the rapid decrease in muscle mass, they simply lack the energy to be active. Sitting all the time decreases metabolic flexibility—as well as joint flexibility. Even if you do manage to get on a treadmill for an hour a day, that intermittent burst of exercise does not overcome the metabolic decrease of sitting around for the other twenty-three hours. A 2013 French study published in the *Journal of Applied Physiology* found that being inactive makes you rely on carbs for quick energy instead of metabolizing stored fat. You wind up converting the incoming sugar into fuel, but if you don't use it immediately, it's then converted into more fat storage in the places it's not supposed to be, like marbled throughout your muscles and liver—the so-called skinny fat effect. Stored fat in your liver and other organs causes oxidation (when your parts turn to rust) and chronic inflammation (when they are puffy and swollen), accelerating cellular death. Your organs, and you, are at high risk for heart disease and cancers.

Dehydration. In the SUNY Stony Brook study mentioned above, the majority of the participants' weight loss wasn't fat. It was water. Quick-energy glucose is stored in muscles with water. Since you lose glycogen (a molecule of stored glucose or sugar) by dieting, water is also released from muscles. Without glycogen and water in your muscles, they appear smaller. Dehydration in muscles modifies your hormonal balance, not in your favor. It increases cortisol, the stress hormone, which encourages the body to hold on to fat cells, especially around your waistline. In effect, water weight loss makes your muscles smaller, keeps them from regrowing, and creates a hostile hormonal environment that bloats your belly. Trust me, dehydration makes muscles weak, no matter how strong you are.

Frankly, I'm surprised the subjects in the SUNY Stony Brook study stuck to the 1,100 calorie diet for the whole eleven weeks. If that isn't unsustainable, I don't know what is. When you're deprived of nutrients by eating so few calories, your body will continually demand nutrients via hunger pangs and cravings. Unless you're eating *very* well, your hunger will go through the roof!

What's more, when your body suspects it's being malnourished, it causes you to crave a quick energy source to save you from dying. Quick-fix cravings mean one thing: junk food. In a 2014 British study, neuroscientists split twenty-two nonobese subjects into two groups. One group was injected with saline; the other with ghrelin, the hormone that causes hunger. After a fasting period, the ghrelin group's hedonistic brain pathways were significantly more stimulated than the saline group's, making them crave high-calorie food. The conclusion: When you're *really* hungry, like on a low-calorie diet, your brain screams, "Eat anything!"

To recap:

Just thinking "diet" is stressful and shifts your brain into deprivation mode, compelling you to eat everything you can get your hands on.

Low-calorie diets only result in water weight loss, which reduces muscles and slows your metabolic rate so much that when you eat normally again, the weight piles on at lightning speed.

You're so weak from self-starvation and dehydration that you refrain from activity and become sedentary, which slows metabolism even more.

When your body is starved of nutrients, it responds by increasing your appetite. Hunger itself causes junk food cravings, which you are too weak from hunger to fight.

The Impact of Too Much Exercise on Metabolism

I know women who work out every day, sometimes twice a day, and still cannot lose fat. It seems counterintuitive, but again, there is an evolutionary imperative at work: In prehistoric times, when we had to hunt and kill our food, we expended energy in necessary bursts. We weren't typically hunting two large mammals a day, every day—there was adequate time to rest and recover before the next hunt. But when you chase that figurative buffalo every single day, your body gets the message: *I really suck at hunting. Better hold on to my fat reserves because I don't know the next time I'll get something to eat.*

Combine overtraining with a very low-calorie diet, and your body not only holds on to fat stores because you are burning through them all the time, but also because it doesn't know when you will replenish the energy you're expending like crazy.

Overtraining, especially without adequate nutrient intake, causes undue stress to your muscles, joints, and endocrine system (a collection of glands around the body that release hormones into the bloodstream sending chemical messages that control the functioning of your organs), affecting performance, mood, and metabolism. Attention CrossFit devotees: Overtraining Syndrome is a real condition, and it dismantles hormonal balance across the board. If you're doing a strenuous workout five or six times a week, you're susceptible.

How do you know if you have Overtraining Syndrome? Here are a few of the symptoms:

Depression. Overtraining compromises important neurotransmitters, including dopamine. The result is a depressed mood and chronic fatigue. You're not sad and tired because your body is spent per se, but because too much exercise actually has a negative impact on your brain function.

Weight gain. Overtraining throws off the delicate interplay between the thyroid, pituitary, and adrenal glands. Optimally, these hormone-producing glands work together in harmony. When they're out of balance, a potential result is hypothyroidism. This causes depression and weight gain plus a bunch of other unsavory symptoms.

A flabby belly and brain. One of the hormones produced by the adrenal glands is cortisol. It floods our brains in response to stress and sets off the fight-or-flight response. When you overtrain, your body is under stress. The result is that your adrenals pump out so much cortisol that they turn into a dry, empty sponge. It's called adrenal depletion, or, in the extreme form, adrenal insufficiency, a major risk factor for depression, poor sleep, poor memory and concentration, low libido, sugar cravings, fatigue, and weight *gain*, especially around the middle. So all that overtraining you're doing to lose the gut can actually add to it.

A common response to not losing fat despite training so hard is to train *even harder*. Once again, it's the worst thing you can do. Non-athletes need to rest for twenty-four hours for every hour of intense training. According to a 2012 internationally led study about Overtraining Syndrome published by the American College of Sports Medicine, even athletes who bust their butt to enhance their performance will actually see their speed and skills decrease if they don't give themselves time to rest and recover. It's the training equivalent of the Law of Diminishing Returns. The harder the athletes work without a break, the worse they perform. This is especially true if you're over thirty. Athletes at this age have told me that the only thing that keeps them competitive is being careful about rest/recovery cycles and proper nutrition.

I'm not saying you can't do CrossFit or train for a triathlon. If there's a specific type of strenuous exercise you love and can't live without, great! With continual endurance training, the body becomes more efficient at converting fat to fuel. Just make sure that you are getting excellent nutrition and ample rest, or your "fun" will not be sustainable long-term. Exercise should improve your endurance, strength, and cardiac capacity. It should give you *more* energy. If it doesn't, then you're overdoing it. Stop working *harder*. Work *smarter* to gain fitness, time, and energy, and to burn fat.

What about Athletes?

It's true that athletes work out in a way that could be technically defined as "overtraining." But serious athletes use intense training to advance their fitness level, not to burn calories or lose weight. They compensate for all of their hours spent exercising by eating large amounts of macronutrients (including plenty of amino acids) and by getting adequate rest. If you ask a pro athlete about the secret to his or her success, I would bet that many would say that proper nutrition and adequate rest are what allow them to recover from an intense workout and get up and do it all over again the next day. Their bodies are metabolic machines that are monitored constantly. They're not eating a low-fat frozen pizza and collapsing into bed for six hours of sleep. If they did, they couldn't be athletes.

For regular exercisers who care as much about weight loss as performance, you should know that resting after workouts boosts fat metabolism. Overtraining causes adrenal depletion. A depleted adrenal gland is incapable of producing human growth hormone (HGH). You need HGH for many reasons, including what is called "afterburn." Afterburn is your body's capacity to continue burning calories post-workout for up to twenty-four hours. Fitness gets the fire going; afterburn is the glowing ember. Now, if you don't have enough muscle-growing HGH in your system during afterburn, your body will consume glycogen in muscles instead of fat. Same thing if you're dehydrated or don't eat enough carbohydrates. It makes no sense when patients exercise to exhaustion—stressing out the adrenal glands—and then refuse to eat a piece of fruit because "all carbs are bad," which only causes the body to hang on to fat. They're running furiously in reverse.

To recap:

Working out excessively without adequate rest and nutrition makes the body hold on to fat for fear that you're never going to catch that buffalo.

Dieting plus overexercising or exercise to compensate for a junk binge causes your muscles, desperate for protein, to consume themselves.

If you work out too much without rest, you will be at risk for depression, weight gain, fatigue, and concentration loss.

What's Your Metabolic Age?

Your basal metabolic rate (BMR) is a measure of how many calories you'd burn if you did nothing but lie in bed all day. A standard BMR calculator (you can easily find one online) will tell you that the BMR for a forty-five-year-old woman at 5'5" and 150 pounds is 1,400 calories per day—meaning, her metabolism will burn 1,400 calories a day just to keep her alive.

The problem with online calculations, though, is that they can't take your body composition into account. If you have a higher ratio of lean muscle mass to fat, your BMR will be higher because muscle is more metabolically active than fat. A professional soccer player who is also 5'5" and weighs 150 pounds will burn more calories just lying around than a similar-size woman with an inverse muscle-to-fat ratio.

Your metabolic age is calculated by comparing your BMR to others in your chronological age group. If you can maintain a high percentage of lean muscle mass, you will have the metabolic rate and age of someone much younger. You'll be more vital, healthier, and stronger with a greater capacity to be active.

As a measure of health and longevity, I prefer metabolic age to real age. Metabolic age is about fitness. If you're forty with the BMR of a twenty-year-old, you will burn more calories than a hot twenty-year-old with no lean muscle mass and the BMR of a forty-year-old. In ten years, that woman is going to look a lot less hot. Or she'll starve herself to stay thin, compromising her fitness, brain, and metabolism. I have seen many women whose bodies look much older than their chronological age because of this. They may still look great in clothes. Naked? They feel devastated by how aged their body appears.

After I lost my sixty pounds of baby weight on the Well Path, I was forty-three years old with the BMR of a seventeen-year-old. I did it one step at a time. I didn't diet. I didn't exercise excessively. I just focused on becoming more fit, nutrifying my body, staying active, and having fun. The weight has stayed off for four years without any sacrifice or feeling of deprivation. I do three yoga classes a week and go hiking whenever I can. I eat whatever I want, which happens to be quality fuel for my hungry body. I haven't counted a calorie or obsessed about weight or ruminated on what's "good" or "bad" in my refrigerator. The Well Path has freed me up to use my energy at work, at home, and in my community.

3

The Truth about Aging

Aging is not a simple calculation of how many years you have existed on the planet. Chronological age is actually just a number, a tally of birthdays that have come and gone. It doesn't reflect your fitness, appearance, ability to fight disease, or your mental sharpness.

We've all met people who seem way younger than their years, and those who seem prematurely withered. I find that the women in my practice who overexercise and chronically diet look much older than their chronological age, as do the women who overeat a nutrient-poor diet. Why? Genes play a big part, of course. Smoking, sun exposure, and anxiety contribute as well. But, by and large, rapid aging is due to stress, both psychological *and* physical. Anything that spins your body out of homeostasis—poor diet, dehydration, lack of rest or sleep, disease, calorie deprivation—causes stress.

Stress opens the door to a host of killer diseases, spurs the accumulation of gunk in your blood vessels and organs, and causes cellular damage and body decay as you rack up the years. Decay isn't a pretty word, but it's accurate. You can slow down the aging process, but not if you're on the hamster wheel of dieting, overeating, freaking out about your weight, and overtraining to compensate for binges or sitting on your butt, disgusted with yourself about your "failure." I feel stressed out just writing this paragraph!

Unless they become sick with cancer or another age-related disease, most women tend not to think that much about what's happening *inside* their body as they get older. Instead, they fixate on the signs of aging they can see in the mirror: the wrinkles, the sun spots, the gray hairs, the sagging skin. They equate "anti-aging" with treatments and procedures to the face or body. The phrases you hear in commercials for anti-aging products are all based on the surface of our bodies: Get "younger-*looking* skin" or "reduce the *appearance* of aging." The products can't go so far as to say "younger skin" and "reduce the speed of aging" because creams and serums can't do that.

I understand the desire to try out the latest anti-aging treatments. Who doesn't want to look younger? I have tried the most potent anti-aging creams and some cutting-edge, noninvasive anti-aging technologies myself, both as research for what to offer at my clinic and, sure, because I hope to find magic in a jar, too. But while these treatments may help you look and feel younger on the outside, they aren't fooling your cells, organs, muscles, and bones.

Frankly, I've observed that even the superficial anti-aging treatments work best when a patient is doing what she can for a healthy internal environment as well. Physiologically, you can fluff up the pillows and comforter over a sagging mattress, but if you do nothing to firm up the mattress itself, you'll always look like a rumpled bed. The surface signs of aging are a clue to what's going on deep inside your body. You must address the internal if you expect to see a difference in the external. Experienced doctors can clue into a patient's diagnosis within one minute of her walking into the exam room, because her appearance sends loud signals about what's happening on the inside.

Yellowing skin might mean liver disease.

A gray tint might indicate heart disease.

Sagging skin or slow-healing wounds might be diabetes.

Cellulite means poor circulation.

Puffy skin might be a thyroid condition.

Dark circles might be allergies.

Rosacea could be an intestinal disorder.

When your skin is in bad shape, it means your internal organs aren't doing so hot, either. It's all connected. Crow's feet won't kill you, but heart disease might.

How We Age

A thirty-second history of the life of a cell: It's born. It joins with other cells of its kind, forming an organ—an eye or a liver or the skin. Each cell contributes to the overall function of its organ for as long as it can. Eventually each individual cell starts to decay, and either it regenerates by copying all of its DNA perfectly and splitting into new baby cells, or it degenerates and dies. Each one of your body's one hundred trillion cells will eventually die. When your cells die faster than others are born, or when your cells become sick and diseased, you, the larger organism, will die. Ever wonder what causes organ failure, or how a heart or liver peters out? It dies, one or more cells at a time.

Ideally, your cells will repair and regenerate at the same rate as they degenerate. In that case, you will stay younger longer. Robust cell health is key throughout your life, but it's especially important after you turn thirty. You can't take cell health for granted once you cross that threshold. You must actively boost cell health to keep your body functioning and on track for a long and vibrant life.

I'm always surprised that people don't connect the fact that their cells need oxygen and nutrients and water to survive, just like we, the larger organism, do. Or that, when a cell gets exposed to too much of a bad thing, it can die like we can. I'm not telling you this to scare you: I'm telling you this to empower you. It's essential to understand how the body ages on a cellular level, so you can make choices that will help you to live as well as you possibly can for as many years as you will have on this planet. And for some reason, the actual story of aging is shrouded in mystery. It's a taboo topic—especially for women.

Just as no substance exists that can make you drop fat like a pile of laundry, there is no magic bullet to reverse the aging process. Our internal systems are intricately intertwined and complex. Yes, nutrition is critical for cell health. Yes, external maintenance, like applying a good-quality moisturizer, can improve the surface pliancy of your skin. But to actually slow the aging process on a cellular level, to grow younger and turn back the clock, you have to get the ebb and flow of your overall physiology in balance. You have to live in a state of homeostasis.

What You're Up Against

After age sixty, your risk of dying doubles every eight years. So the year you turn sixty-eight, you are twice as likely to die as compared to your sixty-year-old friend. Why does the likelihood of death accelerate? The science of aging is evolving, but here are the four factors that we know contribute to the aging process:

Stem cell decline

Shortening telomeres

Glycation

Oxidation stress

Let's take a closer look at each of these factors, and what you can do to help slow down the aging process.

Stem Cell Decline

Stem cells are the source of all new cells in your body. Regular old cells can divide and regenerate for a while, but eventually they die. We need stem cells to give birth to brand-new, bouncing baby cells to replace the old ones.

At birth, stem cells circulate in a baby's bloodstream. New cells are born at an amazing rate, which speeds healing. If a child falls off her bike and breaks her arm, the bones will knit back together in a matter of weeks. She'll be ready for action as soon as the cast comes off.

At thirty-five, stem cell production drops to 55 percent. If you fall off your bike and break your arm, healing will take 45 percent longer. And then, when the cast comes off, you'll have to rehab the atrophied muscles.

At fifty, stem cell production drops to 50 percent. It'll take twice as long to heal that arm, and twice as long to rebuild atrophied muscles as it did a few decades ago. At sixty-five, stem cell production plummets to just 10 percent. At retirement age, it will take months to heal a broken bone. You'll suffer through an extended period of immobility, plus rehab. Aging is a painful, merciless dwindling of your body's once-plentiful resources.

You can't do much about some decline in stem cells over time. It's going to happen. But habits and lifestyle factors like chronic dieting, overtraining, and anxiety have been shown to accelerate the process. Well Path strategies like boosting circulation and nutrifying your cells can help you make the most of the stem cells you have. In the not so distant future, medicine may also offer some interventions for stem cell loss. Right now, practitioners are injecting patients' own stem cells back into their bodies at injury sites or areas with tissue decline for rapid regeneration. The use of exogenously harvested stem cells is an exciting field of research, and it holds great promise for the treatment of many degenerative conditions and diseases.

Shortening Telomeres

Your cells contain your DNA—the genetic information that makes you *you*. Your DNA is made up of chromosomes, which are threads of protein located inside the nucleus of your cells. On the tip of each chromosomal thread is a little protective cap, like the plastic tip on the end of a shoelace. That tip is a telomere.

A cell replicates many times over its life, and when it can't replicate again, it dies. Telomeres regulate cellular replication. They take the brunt of the wear and tear of cell division, and ensure that when your DNA replicates its ends don't become frayed over the years. This is a hugely important responsibility because if your DNA does become damaged in the division process, diseases—such as cancer—can develop. Every time a cell divides to make new cells—about fifty to seventy times in a cell's lifetime—the telomere tip on each chromosome gets progressively shorter. When the telomere can't get any shorter, that cell is done.

If you were genetically blessed with naturally long telomeres, your cells will continue to divide perfectly for a long time, increasing your life span. Geneticist Richard Cawthon of the University of Utah found that his sixty-plus-year-old study subjects who had naturally long telomeres outlived their peers with short telomeres by five years. Cawthon reasoned that if it were possible to lengthen telomeres with behavior, you could add five, ten, or even thirty years to your lifetime.

Well, then, is it possible to keep your telomeres long or even lengthen them?

Indeed it is, by nutrifying your body, balancing activity and rest, and becoming more mindful of sleep and stress.

It's also possible to rapidly shorten them. Here are a few ways your decisions and behavior can contribute to the shortening of your telomeres.

Dieting. A nutrient-poor diet that's low in fiber and antioxidants shortens telomeres. Research has shown that the more fiber you eat, the longer your telomeres can become. In one study, researchers fed subjects a low-protein, high-fiber diet. During the course of the study, the participants' telomeres stretched and their life spans increased.

Thinking about dieting. According to a 2012 study published in the journal *Psychoneuroendocrinology*, researchers put some of their forty-seven overweight female subjects on a wait list for a restrictive eating program. The researchers found that the wait-listed group reported an increase of preoccupation with dieting and eating. During the span of the study, the women's telomeres shrank. The control group, which was not put on a wait list, did not report a preoccupation with dieting and had longer telomeres in the post-study follow-up. The study's conclusion: Anticipating dietary restraint impacts cellular aging.

Chronic stress. In the same study mentioned above, researchers found that the subjects who registered higher levels of cortisol (the "stress" hormone) in their blood serum had decreased telomere length.

A sedentary lifestyle. In a 2008 study published in the *Journal of the American Medical Association*, researchers evaluated the lifestyle of 2,400 volunteers and found that, adjusting for age, smoking, and other habits, the sedentary subjects had shorter telomeres than the ones who were habitually active in their leisure time. The choice between sitting on the couch for hours after work versus taking an after-dinner walk might determine how long and how well you live.

Glycation

When glucose (sugar) binds to proteins and/or fats inside your body as part of the natural metabolic process or outside of it (in the food you eat), a chemical reaction called glycation occurs. Picture a saucepan over high heat. Now, drop in a chunk of butter and watch it melt. Then add a cup of sugar. As the sugar dissolves in the butter and turns into a dark caramel, you are witnessing glycation in action. Sugar (glucose) + butter (fat) + heat = a sweet, sticky goo. When this goo is created in your body or in food, it is known as an advanced glycation end product, or AGE.

AGE couldn't be a more apt acronym. A preponderance of AGEs clog and coat your organs in sticky caramel crud, slowing them down and impairing their ability to function optimally. AGEs are particularly nasty to the collagen and elastin in your skin. The gooey by-products crosslink your skin's proteins, turning springy young skin stiff, wrinkly, and saggy. If you have excessive AGE accumulation in your body, wrinkles are the least of your problems. A diet high in AGEs has been linked to belly fat and insulin insensitivity, bringing you one step closer to diabetes and heart disease. Over time, the buildup can also lead to dementia, renal failure, muscular degeneration, arthritis, and more.

Some glycation can't be avoided. It's a biochemical process, the end result of your body metabolizing sugar. Then there are the AGEs you can avoid: the ones you ingest in foods.

Cooking food using high-temperature methods—such as baking, grilling, broiling, sautéing, and frying—amps up the AGEs. This goes for all foods, even veggies. Grilled chicken, once thought the safest of safe protein options? Not so good for you in terms of AGEs. Grill marks or any other char on food is a signal that it is teeming with the sticky stuff.

According to a 2010 study published in the *Journal of the American Dietetic Association*, reducing dietary AGEs by 50 percent can dramatically lower your risk of developing disease, adding years to your life. You don't have to radically alter your eating habits. No need to sell the backyard grill or throw out your toaster. Just strive for at least one low-AGE meal per day. You don't have to eliminate food groups. Just being mindful of your cooking method and balancing your diet toward low-AGE choices will go a long way toward reducing your AGE exposure.

The further food gets from its natural state, the worse it is for you. Anything made in a factory has been heated with added sugar and fat, and is therefore rife with AGEs.

In their natural state, some food groups have more AGEs than others. Fatty proteins have the most, not surprisingly. Dairy products (milk, cheese, yogurt), which have fat, protein, and sugars, are also high in AGEs, whether they've been heated or not. Melting cheese, for example, adds even more AGEs to it.

Foods that are low in AGEs are those that don't combine sugar and protein/fat. Fruits, raw vegetables, whole grains, unheated healthy oils, like olive and canola, are all great components of a low-AGE meal. Eating a big fresh salad is an easy way to get in a low-AGE meal. Vegetable-based soups or stews are low in AGEs, too.

If you do want to cook your veggies or you're making animal protein, never cook with olive oil! As soon as it hits the hot pan, it's riddled with AGEs. If you must sauté something, do it in coconut oil. If you add a little salt, it cuts the coconut flavor. Or, skip oil and just use water or stock. Crockpot cooking is one of my favorite ways to cook everything I love while minimizing AGEs.

Another way to reduce AGEs in cooked foods is to cook with liquid instead of fire. Slow, wet cooking methods like steaming, boiling, microwaving, poaching, stewing, and souping are great ways to do this. In fact, on the Well Path, you will eat soup every day for lunch. Each recipe includes high-fiber ingredients that have been proven to decrease AGEs. Within a week or two of eating soup for lunch, all of my patients notice changes in the elasticity, color, and firmness of their skin.

Oxidation Stress

Exposure to oxygen causes damage to your body at the cellular level. This damage is known as oxidation stress. Each time you take a breath, oxygen is sent to every cell in your body. During this process, a chemical reaction occurs, creating substances called oxidants. Oxidants can be good for your body, by helping to clean up bacteria, or they can be harmful, by damaging the DNA in your cells.

The buildup of oxidants in your body is progressively corrosive. If glycation clogs your vessels and organs with caramel goo, oxidation turns them to rust. It's the equivalent of leaving a peeled apple on the counter, exposed to air. What happens? The white part oxidizes and turns brown. Metal exposed to air oxidizes and rusts, like the nails in your deck or a car in a junkyard. Rust weakens the structure of metal until, eventually, it disintegrates. In the same way, oxidation breaks down your cells, including the collagen and elastin of your skin cells.

Oxidation *stress* is your body's response to detecting this rust buildup. Your immune system sends in white blood cells to fight it. Blood cells sweep away the bad stuff, but they can't get back out if the vessels and organs are clogged by gooey AGEs. The result is chronic inflammation. In the medical world, we refer to inflamed organs as "hot." A hot colon is the perfect environment for unchecked free radical cells—cells that have an odd number of electrons that try to steal an electron from other, healthy cells, thereby damaging them and possibly causing cancer.

While some degree of oxidation and our body's stress response to it is natural, our habits also have an impact on how much rust we accumulate over the years. Some chief contributing factors to oxidation stress and chronic inflammation: a high-protein, low-fiber diet, stressed-out muscles from overtraining, being sedentary, and being anxious. Notice a pattern?

Our bodies make endogenous antioxidants (ones that exist inside our bodies naturally), but we rely on the exogenous ones—found in food—to do the trick and counterbalance oxidants. Antioxidants are found in a high-fiber diet full of fruit, vegetables, and whole grains. The fiber is like a broom that sweeps away the rust and swelling, and makes you clean and clear and cool on the inside. Guess what? On the Well Path, you will multiply your fiber intake without even thinking about it.

These four components of aging are deeply intertwined. Poor nutrition accelerates stem cell decline and oxidizes your cells. Oxidation stress shortens telomeres. Glycation causes oxidation stress. Glycation also shortens telomeres. You can't combat one without addressing the others. Anti-aging only happens from the outside in. Nothing you can find in a jar, tube, or pill rids you of accumulated AGEs, cools "hot" organs, or sweeps away the rust. The good news is, it's absolutely possible to reverse a rapidly aging state and create a healthy body that will thrive both inside and out. How does that happen? One step at a time.

4

The Truth about Hormones

As you know by now, your endocrine system produces and manages your hormones. Hormones are chemical messengers secreted by glands that enter the bloodstream where they flow throughout the body, washing by every cell. They don't affect every cell they come into contact with, however. In fact, hormones are like keys that fit only into certain locks. The locks are receptor cells on a given organ. When the hormone keys fit into an organ cell's receptor locks, the organ is turned on to perform a particular function. For example, the pancreas secretes insulin into the bloodstream. The insulin key fits into receptors on a muscle cell, unlocking it, which causes glucose to leave the muscle and travel to the liver to be used for energy.

Your hormones are magical. When the right key goes into the right lock, your body will perform just as it should. When the body is in homeostasis, the endocrine system flows effortlessly and works efficiently. In homeostasis, the hormonal system is flexible to respond to the ebb and flow of our physiological needs to keep us in balance.

Unfortunately for most women, their endocrine system is out of whack and inflexible because their body is constantly in a state of reaction instead of homeostasis. When you're under stress, your endocrine glands suppress or flood your body with these chemical keys. The lack or overabundance of hormones, what we call hormonal imbalance, affects how cells behave. Too loud a signal overwhelms cell receptors and the lock stays open for too long. Too faint a signal, and the cell cannot respond fully or stays locked. Sometimes the strength of the signal will even change the normal amount of receptors in your body, making you more or less sensitive to the normal messenger signals. The result of hormonal imbalance is fat retention, oxidation, glycation, inflammation, and cell degeneration, or, in other words, all the things that cause rapid aging and weight gain.

The endocrine system is the most intricate, sensitive, and resourceful system in your body. If I were to draw a schematic of it, it'd be like the New York City subway, Paris metro, and London tube maps tangled up with one another. When it's in balance, this complex system chugs along smoothly. Your body's fifty known hormones work together like dominoes. One tips the other, flowing along in an effortless, natural procession.

When your body is under stress, however, certain hormones are disrupted, which throws off the entire system. Out of balance, your endocrine system is like a mixed-up Rubik's Cube—even when slightly off, it's so hard to put right again. Remember, stress is not limited to the emotional kind, as in "I'm so stressed out right now." Lack of sleep, overtraining, being sedentary, and restrictive dieting are unnecessary layers of stress on the body that make fat loss and optimal functioning a struggle. We evolved to handle fluctuations of stress, but thanks to our hectic modern lives we exist in a state of constant crisis or, at least, that's how our hormones interpret it.

Just to illustrate my point, I'm going to call out a handful of hormones you've probably heard of and explain how they're affected by stress.

Cortisol

The "stress" hormone is released by the adrenal glands when you are under siege (or just think you are), increasing blood sugar to enable the fight-or-flight response. Humans these days aren't running away from buffalos. We're sitting at our desks until late at night, struggling to meet work deadlines. Cortisol brings a sugar flood to provide instant energy. But instead of expending the blood sugar by actually fighting or fleeing, we wind up storing it around our midsections. Eventually, you can become cortisol resistant—your body pumps it out copiously, but you stop reacting to it. You lose the fight-or-flight energy boost, but you keep adding belly fat, suppressing your immune system and puffing up with internal inflammation.

We usually think of stress as something that happens to us. And, certainly, there is stress that we cannot control, like a death in the family, the loss of a job, or taking care of an ailing parent. But then there is the stress that we bring on ourselves. A sedentary person who sits at her desk all day is under stress. A mom who's shuttling three kids around all day and doesn't have time to eat well or exercise is also under stress. If you can learn to balance emotional and physical stress with healthy habits—good nutrition, adequate rest, reasonable activity levels—you'll lose excess belly fat and regain cortisol sensitivity.

Dopamine

This hormone is often described as the "feel good" or "reward" hormone. When you do something thrilling, like fall in love, ride a roller coaster, have sex, or take drugs, your brain gets a hit of this chemical. Not surprisingly, it is possible to become addicted to dopamine, leading you to repeat the same thrill-seeking behavior to get another hit. Eating comfort food when under stress is one way to get it. According to an article in the *Journal of Neuroscience*, the more you eat to relieve stress, the deeper the dopamine neural pathways become and the harder it is to stop the habit.

Most of us associate certain foods with emotions or memories. You might equate a milkshake with a special childhood tradition—maybe your mom would treat you to one when you were upset. As an adult, when you're lonely or upset, a milk shake—and the quick hit of dopamine it releases—makes you feel better. Your brain learns to associate that food with a hormonal reward, and that pathway is reinforced each time you reach for a milk shake. But, like with cortisol, you can become insensitive to too much dopamine. Receptors get overwhelmed and start to shut down, blocking the ability of the hormone to function properly. Soon you need more, bigger milk shakes to get the same hit of calming maternal love.

The only way to change this behavior is to forge new neural pathways and make new, healthier associations. On the Well Path, you'll do this by eating a wide variety of nutritious foods, including soups—the ultimate comfort food. At the end of an eight-week Path, my patients call me and say, "What am I going to do without the soups?" They've swapped their stress-eating addiction for healthy eating, which isn't a bad addiction to have.

Comfort Food Creates Hormonal Havoc

Heather, forty-three, put on about twenty pounds when her father was ill and couldn't get rid of the extra weight. "I'd visit him in the hospital. There was an ice cream place across the street. Once a week, I'd get a chocolate malt as a little treat. Then I'd get a small chocolate malt every day. Then I started getting a large malt every day. I felt lost that my dad was dying. I lost any feeling of control," she said.

It wasn't discipline she was up against. Drinking the malts released dopamine into her brain's reward center. She came to associate the sadness of seeing her sick father with the reward of a chocolate malt. The neural pathways formed quickly, and she became addicted. It's a classic case of feeding uncomfortable sensations, not hunger, and becoming hooked on it.

And, with care and awareness, you can become unhooked. After a month on the Well Path, Heather came back to see me, bubbling with excitement. Years ago, she'd had T-shirts made with her business logo on them. After she gained weight, she couldn't fit into them. She gestured at her chest, proudly exclaiming, "I'm wearing my shirt!"

Ghrelin

When your stomach is empty and your body needs nutrients, ghrelin tells the brain, "Feed me!" If you combine ghrelin with dopamine—by responding to hunger with a milk shake—you'll crave junk in response to hunger instead of healthy food that will provide the nutrients your body is actually craving. You don't want to combine cortisol and ghrelin, either. In a 2013 study published in the journal *Behavioral Brain Research*, scientists observed that there was a dynamic interplay between ghrelin and cortisol. The more stress their obese female subjects experienced, the more hunger they experienced. The conclusion drawn was *not* that being obese makes it harder to cope with stress, but that difficulty coping with stress makes your hunger hormone go nuts. As a result, you cannot resist your body's desire for food.

Growth Hormone

Human growth hormone, or HGH, produced by the pituitary gland, stimulates cell growth and regeneration, repairs skin, and metabolizes fat. Fat cells contain HGH receptors and are just waiting to be unlocked by this hormone. HGH also helps to build muscle and convert glucose into energy. We like HGH. You want lots of it in your system for fat loss and cell regeneration. Unfortunately, aging and bad habits cause HGH to decline sharply. For example, if you eat lots of carbs (perhaps on a low-fat diet), you won't have enough HGH to unlock fatty acids from fat cells. That's because insulin (more on this hormone in a minute) and HGH are on a seesaw. When one goes up, the other goes down. Since HGH is only produced while you're sleeping, sleep deprivation drives down production. Another HGH suppressor is sporadic, medium-duration, medium-intensity exercise, like putting in forty-five minutes on the treadmill, in an otherwise sedentary existence.

Insulin

When you eat sugar, your pancreas releases insulin, a hormone intended to guide the incoming glucose to the liver to be converted to glycogen, a form of quick fuel that is used by your muscles when they need energy. But when you consume too much glucose—like eating a bagel followed by a doughnut at brunch—your insulin levels spike, and your body can't handle the influx. Some of that glucose goes to the muscles, but the rest of it is sent to fat cells for long-term storage. Over time and a ton of doughnuts, you can become insulin resistant. Instead of getting a sugar rush of instant energy, your confused insulin receptors send all the sugar into your fat cells, making you feel sluggish and, tragically, ravenous for more sugar, which you *can't stop eating*. Which brings us directly to . . .

Leptin

Leptin is produced in your fat cells. Its job is to signal your brain when you feel satiated from a meal. Leptin is supposed to say, "I'm full now, please stop eating." If you have a lot of fat cells, leptin should be even more sensitive and signal you even more quickly. But two things disrupt leptin's regulatory functions: eating too much and, in particular, eating too much sugar. Eating too much sugar causes insulin resistance, which, in a roundabout but predictable way, leads to leptin resistance. Fat cells fill up as a result of eating sweets, and, at the same time, the trigger that would slow down that process is muffled. Bingeing turns off the switch that says one Cronut is enough. Ironically, fasting does the same thing. Eating a too-low-calorie diet decreases leptin sensitivity. The less you eat, the hungrier you feel. Makes sense. Your body thinks you're starving. It has no idea you're just on some weird cleanse. So, when the cleanse is over and you start eating again, leptin is still stunned and doesn't get the memo to wake up anytime soon. For example, if you dieted in anticipation of Thanksgiving, you will stuff yourself like a turkey, over and over again. This is how you can gain five pounds over one long weekend.

Melatonin

The "drowsy" hormone regulates our sleep/wake cycle. When darkness falls, melatonin spikes and we begin to feel drowsy. When the sun rises, melatonin drops and we wake up. This cycle is known as your circadian rhythm. In recent years, our plugged-in lives have made it a lot tougher for melatonin to do its job. As a result of constant exposure to glowing screens, melatonin levels constantly fluctuate, disrupting normal circadian rhythms. Insomnia is a common problem in America, and I often see it among my patients.

Not getting enough sleep impacts your overall health, including your eating habits. Anxiety-related insomnia has an impact on the enzymes in your bowels that break down food. So lack of sleep actually interferes with how well your gut absorbs nutrients. Poor absorption makes you crave more food to make up for nutrient deficits. Your metabolic rate also downshifts if you get less than seven hours of sleep a night because your body believes it's in crisis and hangs on to energy stores.

Keeping your screens on past sundown in the winter is especially harmful, because our bodies are programmed to store fat during the summer, in times of plenty, and are signaled to do so by the extra daylight. Too much exposure to light in the winter will prompt your body to store even more fat.

Last and worst, sleep deprivation boosts the production of "feed me!" ghrelin and decreases "I'm full" leptin. In numerous studies, people who get less than seven hours of sleep per night have been found to have a higher BMI than people who get a good night's sleep.

Phenylethylamine

Phenylethylamine, or PEA for short, is a neurotransmitter in the brain that, like dopamine, makes you feel good. It's a natural stimulant—your body's own version of speed—and is responsible for giddy feelings, like the initial rush of falling in love. PEA is found in chocolate, a fact that may help explain why women tend to crave it when they're stressed out, upset, and off balance. It's also found in blue-green algae, which I've been supplementing my diet with for fifteen years and credit with keeping me on an even keel emotionally, despite my hectic life.

Low levels of PEA are associated with neurological health issues, such as ADHD and depression. In a recent study, researchers at Rush University and the Center for Creative Development in Chicago gave small doses of PEA to fourteen patients who'd had major depressive episodes. Almost a year later, twelve of the subjects reported a significantly improved mood and were still responding to the treatment. But you don't need to take a supplement or eat a chocolate bar to get a boost of this important hormone—you just need to go for a run. In fact, when researchers at Nottingham Trent University in England asked a group of men to run on a treadmill for thirty minutes and then measured their PEA levels, they found that PEA increased in 90 percent of the men post-exercise. What this means for you: Being sedentary is a surefire way to feel unhappy—and that unhappiness can lead to depression and weight gain. On the Well Path, we will make your mental health just as much of a focus as your physical health—and you will see that you can't have one without the other!

Reproductive Hormones

Imbalances of estrogen, progesterone, prolactin, testosterone, and other reproductive hormones are responsible for PMS and menopause symptoms, as well as certain cancers, including breast cancer. Many women have told me that their PMS and/or menopause symptoms improved on the Well Path. I didn't set out to cure either set of symptoms, but I'm so pleased that the program can offer these benefits! It's not clear why these results were possible for them, but one recent study (conducted in India in 2014) suggests that regular exercise may be the magic bullet. In this study, scientists divided one hundred women into two groups, one that exercised and one that didn't, and then monitored their PMS symptoms. The exercisers reported fewer PMS symptoms than the non-exercisers. It is believed that aerobic workouts balanced reproductive hormones, making the week before menstruation a smoother ride.

Postmenopausal women shouldn't feel left out of the benefits, either. When estrogen levels decline, you are less efficient at using fat for fuel during exercise. But the good news is that you can increase estrogen—as well as testosterone—with strength training. Increasing muscle mass will also strengthen bones, a major health concern as we get older.

Decreasing estrogen and progesterone—in the latter two weeks of your menstrual cycle and during perimenopause and menopause—also impacts digestion by causing a slowing of intestinal movement. This slowing alone may cause changes in intestinal flora, which will affect the absorption of nutrients and boost appetite. When estrogen is very low—in menopause—cortisol levels rise, which slows the release of stomach acid. It takes longer to empty your intestine and brings on gas, bloating, and constipation. So your appetite is bigger and your digestion is less efficient.

As you eat more fiber on the Well Path, those issues will be tamed, and you'll lose weight, which, in turn, lowers your risk of breast cancer. In 2012 in the *Journal of Clinical Oncology*, an international team of researchers reported the results of their yearlong study of overweight postmenopausal women ages fifty to seventy-five. As the subjects lost weight by eating balanced diets and exercising, their serum levels of estrogen and free testosterone decreased, lowering their biomarkers for breast cancer.

As you can see, our delicate hormonal system is vitally important to our overall health. One hormonal imbalance causes a fifty-car pileup on the biochemical superhighway. It's not humanly possible to boost or reduce the release of one hormone or another without throwing others out of balance. The body has developed in an exquisite way to survive and thrive. Stress and dieting upset your hormonal balance. In order to lose weight and age well, we need to allow our hormones to function the way they were designed to, and not stress about targeting individual hormones. The best you can do is shoot for balance and flexibility. And the good news is that your body will do all of this for you if you treat it well. Finding that balance, that sweet spot, is the goal of the Well Path.

The next section in this book explains how you'll do just that, and get your body back to homeostasis. Real, meaningful, sustainable change is possible when you follow the Well Path.

PART TWO

The Well Path

5

Getting in Balance

Over the next two months, you'll gently nudge your body back into homeostasis and reap the rewards. You'll swap fat for muscle, nutrify your cells, and balance hormones for sounder sleep and hotter sex.

How can such dramatic change happen so quickly? Some of my patients don't believe it's possible, but then again, they've been influenced by their previous disappointments with diet and exercise plans that didn't live up to their promises. But I can assure you that change *is* possible. On the Well Path, it's inevitable. Sustainable change is the heart and soul of my wellness philosophy. The categories of C.H.A.N.G.E. are the paving stones of the Path.

C is for Circulation. A congested and stagnant circulatory system prevents stored fat from being used as energy, traps excess fluids where you don't want them, and bathes your cells in harmful oxidants. A wide-open vascular and lymphatic highway flushes away toxins, mobilizes fat, and rushes nutrients and oxygen to hungry cells. On the Well Path, you will get your circulation flowing like a mighty river.

H is for Hunger/Hormone Balance. Chronic dieters and stress eaters are hypersensitive to hunger pangs. They don't know the difference between real and false hunger, which causes panicked overeating or cravings for calorie-dense junk food. On the Path, you'll become aware of your triggers, learn how to distinguish between real and false hunger pangs, and discover strategies to end stress eating.

A is for Activity. Sitting is the new smoking. Boosting non-exercise activity (movement that doesn't cause sweating) increases metabolism and circulation and can burn an additional 400 calories a day. You'll slowly increase activity to get blood flowing to the dead-end zones, metabolize stored fat from all over your body, and boost your fat-burning ability during exercise.

N is for Nutrition. Our bodies need it all—carbs, fat, protein, micronutrients, and fiber. On the Path, you won't be eliminating *any* food groups, including brownies. You'll nutrify what you already love by adding the Four F's—fruit, fat, fiber, and fuel (protein)—to your favorite meals. In doing so, you'll improve gut absorption, decrease hunger, balance hormones, activate cell repair, and speed up metabolism.

G is for General Health. To be all-around healthy, strengthen the four pillars of wellness: sleep, sex, stress management, and social interaction. Each one of the Four S's of optimal health does incredible things for your body and mind, including speeding up your metabolism to get rid of excess fat, boosting cell repair to slow aging, and strengthening your immune system.

E is for Exercise. Exercise improves every system of the body—if done the right way. Typical gym workouts increase stress and consume muscle, not fat. They feel like a self-imposed punishment. On the Path, you'll do fun fitness three or four times a week.

C.H.A.N.G.E. is a pretty perfect mnemonic, isn't it? I remember the day I thought of it. I was walking through Central Park toward my office, thinking about all the necessary steps it takes to get from "nothing works" to homeostasis. I thought, *Well, for starters, you need a vibrant circulation. But you have to exercise and be active, too. Exercise can't compensate for overeating, so hunger has to be sorted out, which is impossible unless you get a decent night's sleep. If you're too busy to sleep, see friends, or have sex, stress goes through the roof. And then there's the lack of fiber in the American diet and all those starved cells . . .* Everything I know about optimal health, weight loss, and anti-aging fit into large categories—Circulation, Activity, Hunger. The words appeared in my mind, and then the acronym shifted into place. It truly was like a lightbulb went on in my head that day on the footpath.

Yes, I thought of C.H.A.N.G.E. while literally putting one foot in front of the other on an actual path.

I'd been working with patients on these strategies for years already, but until that morning I hadn't put them all together in such a systematic way. That day, I started talking to patients about the principles of C.H.A.N.G.E., and then the signposts and map of the Well Path crystallized. It has worked wonders with my patients, and if you commit to change it will work for you, too.

Change is what you want; C.H.A.N.G.E. is how you'll get it.

6

Circulation

What exactly is your circulatory system and why is it so crucial for fat loss and healthy aging?

You know that blood moves through your arteries, veins, and capillaries, supplying oxygen and nutrients to every cell of your body. Along with the nutrients that enter your bloodstream through your digestive system and the oxygen that enters through your pulmonary system, liberated fat from your fat cells enters your bloodstream via tiny vessels interspersed among your fat stores.

The order of operations:

The fat cells get a message that the body needs energy.

Free fatty acids (FFAs) and glycerol, a sugar molecule, are liberated from the fat cells, making the cells shrink. It's just like letting air out of a balloon.

FFAs and glycerol (now liberated fat) are mobilized via the bloodstream and sent to the liver.

The fat is metabolized by your liver and sent to the cells that need energy.

And last, the liberated energy is consumed.

Fat liberation is a natural part of being alive, but it is increased by exercise and activity because your body senses a need for energy. Step two in the process—mobilizing the fat—depends upon a widespread and robust circulatory system. If FFAs can't get into the bloodstream to start their journey to being consumed, they are slurped right back into the fat cells.

When I was in medical school, we had to dissect several corpses. One of mine was of a morbidly obese woman. When I opened her abdomen, I had to cut through masses of yellow, globular belly fat. As I carefully removed the fat that encased the organs, I examined the yellow masses very closely. I couldn't find any healthy-looking blood vessels. All I could see were disproportionately small and weak blood vessels in and among the fat lobules.

When this woman's body sensed a need for energy, her fat cells would have leaked FFAs and glycerol. Even if she were doing everything "right," I couldn't see how the fat would have been mobilized. It was trapped. If this woman had come to me when she was alive, I would have emphasized improving her circulation as strongly as nutrition and physical activity.

Circulation is the crux of our existence. Cells thrive when they get optimal delivery of oxygen and nutrients. Cells falter when they're starved and left to stew in their own waste. Circulation is crucial. It's critical. It's a coincidence that C is the first letter in C.H.A.N.G.E., but it *is* the first step toward homeostasis. Weight loss and anti-aging can't begin until you open up and stretch your vessels to every nook and cranny in your body, especially to "dead-end" areas. Your cells will be able to function optimally, and the leaky fat cells can shrink when your circulatory system whisks away liberated fat.

Your skin also suffers when your circulatory system isn't as robust as it should be. Liposuction offers a great example of what happens to the skin and underlying structures when circulation is compromised. While the procedure is known for vacuuming out fat, it also vacuums out blood vessels. As a result, the overlying skin in the affected area can't get the nutrients it needs to bounce back, making it sag and pucker. Cellulite actually gets worse after liposuction because the destruction to the circulation decreases the delivery of oxygen and nutrients to your skin, and also causes stagnation of lymph. The resulting buildup of free radicals and oxidation degrades the collagen and elastin necessary for healthy, youthful skin.

There is a secondary part of your circulatory system that is distinct from, but connected to, your bloodstream—your lymphatic system. Blood is pumped by your heart at high pressure through your vessels. When it gets to small capillaries, some fluid is squeezed out. That fluid is called lymph. Its main job is to sweep up toxins and cellular waste.

Patients often ask, "What is cellular waste?"

As a whole organism, you take in food, water, and oxygen, and then you excrete stool, urine, sweat, and saliva. Humans are waste creators. Now, zoom in to a single cell. It takes in nutrients and oxygen. After it "eats," it creates waste, too. Cellular waste from every cell in your body goes into your lymphatic system. Before "dirty" lymph rejoins the bloodstream, the cellular waste and environmental/dietary toxins are filtered out by your kidneys, liver, and intestines. Cellular waste leaves your body the same way human waste does—you excrete it.

If blood brings the picnic, lymph cleans up after.

Your lymphatic system does not have a heart that pumps the fluids along at a steady pace. Slow-moving or stagnant lymph gets trapped in the spaces between cells. It can become a cesspool for toxins and waste. You don't want that sitting around in your body for long periods of time. Lymph buildup causes oxidation stress, hormonal imbalance, and shortened telomeres, all three of the rapid aging factors. You can see evidence of these waste-and-toxin puddles on the surface of your skin: the bloating and dimpling, otherwise known as cellulite. There is no real mystery to cellulite. It is simply the result of stagnant fluid retention plus toxins and cell waste. To add insult to injury, stagnant lymph breaks down collagen and elastin. Hence, the loose skin on your thighs.

When our ancestors were on their feet all day hunting and gathering, their circulatory systems were moving freely. Our sedentary lifestyle of spending hours at a time at our desks, followed by hours sitting on the couch, is the equivalent of putting up multiple road blocks and detours on our circulation highway. What should be eight lanes of free-flowing traffic turns into two lanes with maddening congestion. For good health, you have to get *nutrients in* and *waste out*. Opening up more lanes of your circulatory superhighway enables you to do just that.

I live in New York City, and occasionally we have garbage strikes. The trash piles up on the curb, and after a few days, it starts to really stink. Bugs and rats feed on the garbage and soon rotting garbage is strewn everywhere. You can practically see the disease in the air. But when the trucks arrive again and take away the trash, the smell gets better. Bugs go away. Flowers bloom and kids play on the sidewalk.

Blocked circulation is like a garbage strike inside your body. A healthy circulation system is like the garbage man coming each day to take the trash away, leaving your body as healthy and clean on the inside as you will soon see reflected on the outside.

"My Yoga Butt Has Cellulite!"

A common complaint. Patients say, "I exercise, I'm active. I have toned muscles. So why do I still have cellulite?" Their butts are just not getting oxygen and nutrients, and lymphatic drainage is stagnant due to sitting for long periods of time. If you do yoga once a day, but sit on your tush for the other waking hours, cellulite and loose skin are going to happen.

Cellulite has nothing to do with muscle tone. You could have powerful buns of steel with some cottage cheese dimples on top.

Exercise does get circulation moving. However, forty-five minutes of cardio doesn't necessarily increase blood flow to *every* part of your body throughout the day. You heart will pump blood only through wide and adequate blood vessels. But the dead-end zones with inadequate vasculature? They're still going to struggle, especially as we get older and our circulation diminishes naturally.

Cardio does not increase circulation to and through subcutaneous fat, the wiggle bits on top of muscles. Belly rolls, saddlebags, and love handles are meant for emergency storage and are supposed to be hard to access. I have patients who say that their faces turn bright red when they exercise, but their bellies stay cold to the touch. If your vascular highway is closed or nonexistent, exercise and diet can't help you. The good news is, you can stretch and strengthen your circulation. It starts as simply as brushing your teeth. Just keep reading. . . .

So how can you expand your circulation to every nook and cranny of your body, including the dead-end zones? You have to move that blood and lymph. Straggly vessels don't get stronger or more profuse unless you take steps to make them that way. Most of the high-tech machines I use in my practice stimulate new blood vessel growth. But you can accomplish it with low-tech, inexpensive yet effective methods, too. My strategies might, at first, seem insubstantial, but before long, you'll realize how much of a difference they make. This is true for all of the strategies on the Well Path. They may seem too good to be true and too easy to do, but, cumulatively, the small steps of C.H.A.N.G.E. bring on dramatic results.

How to Boost Circulation

Strategies you'll use on the Well Path include:

Drink Warm Lemon Water Each Morning

First thing in the morning, before you eat anything, drink a big mug or two of hot water with fresh lemon juice. If you weigh less than 150 pounds, use half a lemon. If you weight more than 150, use the whole lemon.

The water is hydrating. Hydration in and of itself boosts circulation and gets fluids moving faster through the body. Picture a trickle through a drainpipe versus an overflowing gutter. A big glass of water in the morning instead of dehydrating coffee will make you feel like a dewy fresh rose.

Whenever heat is near a blood vessel, it opens and expands. Drinking hot water before your first bite of food increases blood flow to your gastrointestinal system, preparing it to absorb the nutrients you put in afterward.

The lemon has many wonderful properties that are beneficial for digestion, pH balance, nutrition, and detoxification, and it makes your hot water taste great.

Breathe Deeply

Yogis are familiar with pranayama breathing, the practice of breathing deeply into your diaphragm. Deep breathing can bring up to ten times more oxygen into your bloodstream than normal shallow breathing. The rhythmic contraction and compression of your diaphragm acts as a pump to move lymph along and opens up valves to get the flow going. Deep breathing has also been proven to lengthen telomeres, boost the immune system, balance the hypothalamic-pituitary-adrenal axis, and reduce stress. You can improve circulation and halt aging in the time it takes to inhale.

On the Well Path, you'll try two variations of deep breathing:

Morning pranayama wakes up your body. I recommend practicing this first thing in the morning, before you get out of bed, as it will get your blood flowing after a long night's rest. Here's how to do it: Lying on your back, inhale deeply through the nose, pushing your belly out. When you can't take in any more air, slowly exhale through the mouth, drawing your abdomen in, compressing your lungs. That's the basic rhythm. For five minutes each morning, practice pranayama breathing and combine it with isolated muscle contractions. Starting at your extremities and working steadily toward your center mass, clench one muscle with your inhale, and unclench with your exhale. Contracting your muscles facilitates blood flow. Relaxing them allows the blood to get into your muscles, brain, and tissues throughout your body. With daily practice, you should be able to fill your lungs all the way into the space behind your clavicles.

You will also practice deep breathing before going to sleep at night. Nighttime pranayama is for relaxation, using the same technique minus the muscle contractions.

Dry Brush

You brush your teeth and your hair every day. But did you know that you should also brush your skin every day? Skin brushing stimulates the lymphatic system, increases blood circulation, exfoliates, improves skin tone, and aids kidney and digestive function. Once you have a proper brush (the most you would spend on one at Amazon is $20, but you can get one at any drugstore for around $7), start dry brushing in the morning or in the evening before bed (for detailed instructions, see page 176). If possible, drink a big glass of water immediately afterward to help flush out the toxins you've dislodged. I'm addicted to dry brushing. I do it twice a day, once in the morning and once before bed. My dry brush lives next to my toothbrush, so it's right there and ready to go. It takes less than five minutes and is so worth it. A fifty-year-old patient of mine said her cellulite had vanished after dry brushing twice a day for a couple of months!

Get Upside Down

To counteract those hours of sitting, where your legs are positioned below your heart and not involved in muscular activity, you will spend a few minutes a day getting your legs above your heart, letting gravity do the work of draining them passively. Yogis know this practice as "legs up the wall." You'll start doing these inversions at Week Four on the Path. For more details on how to practice leg inversions, turn to page 188.

Take Hot-Cold-Hot Showers

Hot showers dilate the superficial blood vessels to your periphery. Cold showers constrict the vessels and force the blood back into your core to keep your internal organs warm. Exposing your skin to hot and then cold water is like exercise for your circulatory system. Hot/cold showers are a great way to keep circulation in tip-top condition. Going back and forth between temperatures gets your blood zooming all over your body. Here's what to do: Get in the shower and turn it on as hot as you can stand it for as long as you can. Then switch to as cold as you can stand it for as long as you can. Then back to hot. It'll be challenging at first. You don't have to go ice cold, just turn the temperature down, with the goal of getting colder each time. Eventually, you will crave the incredible sensation you feel from the alternating hot and cold.

Pregnant women or those trying to become pregnant: Skip hot/cold showers until you are safely through your first trimester. After that, don't make the water temperature too hot. Don't go more than five degrees hotter than your ordinary preference. You can go ten degrees colder, though.

Go into Hot and Cold Rooms

Heat widens blood vessels. It's why your face turns red in a Jacuzzi. Hot rooms of 100 degrees F or more force the body to consume energy (free fatty acids and glucose) at a faster rate. If you have access to a hot room, like a sauna or hot yoga studio, use it.

Cold rooms of 66 degrees F or lower stimulate the production of brown fat. This is a good thing. Your body has two kinds of fat: white and brown. White fat is energy storage and accumulates in your belly, thighs, and butt. Brown fat accumulates in your upper chest and shoulders and actually boosts energy consumption. It stimulates your metabolism to burn the lipids in white fat to keep your body warm. If you can lower your white fat and increase brown fat, your metabolism will speed up. People with more brown fat are thinner, have an easier time losing weight, and maintain weight loss better than those with more white fat. Studies have shown that if you keep your thermostat in the 62-to-66-degree F range, you can shift the balance of white and brown fat in your favor. Low 60s sounds cold, I know. If you lower the thermostat progressively, it's easier to take. I nudged mine down to 65 degrees F, which was tolerable. After two weeks, I moved it to 62. I don't even feel the coolness anymore. The kids complain, and I just tell them to wear socks and a sweater. They'll thank me when they're full of brown fat! (Actually, they probably won't. Frowns.) Plus, turning down your thermostat has been shown to help you sleep better.

Pregnant women or those trying to become pregnant: Don't use Jacuzzis, steam rooms, or saunas throughout your pregnancy. Feel free to lower your thermostat. You're probably overheating anyway and have already turned it down.

Get a Massage

I don't like to recommend a strategy that costs more than a few dollars. But if you can afford it, get a massage once a month. A massage is best done the week before the onset of your menstrual cycle, if that's when you retain fluid. Lymphatic drainage massages specialize in the wavelike motion that gets stagnant lymph rolling. But any massage will do. For treatments that have intrinsic cost, my philosophy is to do as much as you can afford in terms of time and money, but not at all if it adds stress to your life. If you can get monthly massages, time them to coincide with the week of your cycle when you have the most water retention. If you no longer have a cycle, the best timing is immediately after vigorous physical activity in order to mobilize the fluid that sometimes accumulates after a workout. The quicker you get rid of it, the better. Self-massage or partner massage is just as good.

Soon enough, you'll actively stimulate circulation using these methods. Start slowly so you're not overwhelmed, adding strategies each week. Studies have shown that by increasing your blood flow regularly, angiogenesis—the process by which baby blood vessels are born—will be stimulated. Picture your insides like that clean city street, with the flowers blooming and kids running around under a blue sky . . . and the sweet smell of success.

High-Tech Options

Everyone can improve their circulation by using the strategies I described in this chapter. The more you do, the better the results. By the end of the sixty days, these strategies will become second nature to you.

In my practice, I use a few high-tech machines to improve circulation to dead-end areas. Technology is a powerful tool to boost circulation. The ones I describe below are a great option for women who have the resources. I find that they are particularly useful for anyone who has had liposuction and has very poor circulation.

Vacuum suction. Suction machines use a handheld head attached to, essentially, a vacuum. The device head has rollers on it. As you roll the device over the top layer of skin with the vacuum on, your skin is gently massaged. This suction and rolling motion forces blood to the surface of the skin. Your brain gets the message that the area needs more blood flow. Eventually, vessels will expand or grow to meet the demand. This is why patients have to keep coming in until circulation improves. You can't grow blood vessels overnight. Some patients come in with very poor circulation to their lower bodies. When I first vacuum their backsides, the skin doesn't even turn pink and is crepe-paper thin. It improves with repeated treatments.

Carboxy Therapy. This is the most effective and cost-efficient treatment I offer. I have a machine that delivers CO_2 (carbon dioxide, the stuff we exhale) to dead-end areas via acupuncturelike needles inserted into the subcutaneous fat layer anywhere on a patient's body. CO_2 causes the blood flow to accelerate to that area by dilating the vessels. This increased flow of oxygen into a poorly circulated area, when done repeatedly, signals the body to generate new blood vessels there, enhancing the circulation long-term.

7.

Hunger

Hunger is a survival instinct. If we didn't feel hunger—stomachs rumbling, thoughts fixated on acquiring food—we wouldn't be compelled to feed our bodies the nutrients we need to live. Hunger is one of the first survival instincts we experience after we're born. It's also one of our strongest instincts, way stronger than sex (but maybe that's just a mother of three talking). On an evolutionary level, hunger is our best friend. Without it, we would die.

Women are bedeviled by hunger when they try to master it. If hunger were a simple case of mind over matter, it'd be easy to control. But when your stomach is empty and every cell in your brain and body is clamoring for nourishment, your willpower is as feeble as a newborn kitten. Add to that the slew of external triggers—signs, TV commercials, magazine covers, pop-up ads—that call out to us at every turn, reminding us of all the delectable options within reach. Add to that the everyday uncomfortable sensations that trigger hunger—stress, sadness, boredom, fatigue—and send you to the fridge. (No one eats excessively because they're full of joy.) Add to *that* the guilt of overeating or "cheating," despite the multitude of internal and external forces that compel you to eat.

That's a lot to go up against.

Hunger *should be* a survival instinct. But due to the combination of these factors, it feels like friction to your psyche, a stab in the belly, and a source of guilt, shame, and regret. For most women, hunger doesn't feel like a healthy, natural impulse. It feels like the enemy.

First and foremost, let me assure you that *true* hunger is such a deep physiological urge that you cannot overcome it with willpower. Why we try to do so baffles me. The very second you "tell" your body it's going to enter a state of deprivation, it *instinctively* becomes hungry and will seek out food, any food. It is impossible to overcome the strength of this instinct. Do not try!

"There must be a pill, right?" my patients often ask me. "What about açai berries or green coffee beans?" Women are only too willing to "try everything" to curb their appetites. I don't recommend these products in my practice because the sensation of true hunger should never be suppressed, and the other sensations that compel you to eat to alleviate discomfort should be acknowledged and distinguished from the sensation of true hunger. The natural instinct of our body is to take in what we need and be satisfied and not seek more. Knowing when you're hungry and when you're full is the magic pill you need to get back to. This is hunger homeostasis.

The only way to truly control hunger is to not try to control it.

I know that sounds annoyingly paradoxical. Give me the next few pages to explain how hunger works, and you'll understand what I mean.

How Your Body Signals Hunger

As you know, our hormones regulate our appetite. They turn on our digestive systems and determine whether our calories are stored or burned. More than a dozen hormones govern our appetites and digestion, but I'm going to focus on the two we've already discussed: ghrelin, which is released by the stomach and makes it rumble when it's empty, and leptin, which is released by your fat cells and signals "I'm full" to the brain.

These hormones work in tandem. In homeostasis, their cues are clear and resonant. Think of your naturally thin friends who never diet or worry about their appetite. I would wager that they wait to eat until ghrelin is released and stop eating when leptin kicks in. They make it look so easy. But for them, it truly is. They allow their hormones to regulate their eating habits without getting in the way. Chronic dieting, fasting, or overeating makes hunger hormones go haywire. You genuinely don't know if and when you're truly hungry or full and wind up eating in response to emotions and other cues.

When you restrict food, depriving your body of adequate calories or a particular nutrient, your stomach pumps out ghrelin by the boatload, screaming "Feed me!" to the hypothalamus in your brain. If you don't respond with food, hunger will increase exponentially. Your body just won't tolerate being denied energy. Before long, even the most determined dieter is hormonally compelled to eat the wallpaper off the walls. The tragic part is that ghrelin levels don't drop after you give in. They continue to pump copiously, as if you were still dieting, for up to a year. It's a lose-lose equation. You might starve weight off, but your hormones will make you pay for it with severe hunger and cravings *for months* afterward. No wonder 90 percent of dieters gain all the weight back in that time frame.

Meanwhile, leptin goes similarly off the rails. The amount of leptin in your bloodstream is determined by your existing fat stores. As I've mentioned before, thin people have less of it, so the "full" signal is faint and takes longer to sound. Heavier people have more, so the signal is louder and goes off quickly, but chronic cycles of deprivation and overeating cause the brain to stop registering it.

You must have heard the line: "I might as well stick that cupcake right on my butt, because that's where it'll show up tomorrow." If a woman has imbalanced hunger hormones, this isn't a joke: it's a fact.

I know I've painted a bleak picture of appetite. But the news isn't all bad. It is possible to reset your hunger hormones. You can undo the damage, step by step, meal by meal, thought by thought. On the Well Path, you'll come to understand hormonal hunger triggers and respond to them appropriately. You'll relearn what empty and full feel like.

How Your Brain Thinks about Hunger

Hunger isn't only a physiological phenomenon. It's psychological, too.

I reflexively bristle when I hear patients say, "I feel fat." I grew up in the '70s and '80s, when awareness of eating disorders became headline news in this country. I watched all of those after-school specials. They taught us to separate weight from emotion. Easy to say, hard to do. As a culture, we continue to send a message to women that the number on the scale determines their value as a person. I know some women who weigh themselves twice a day, and a one- or two-pound difference determines their outlook for the entire day. What a waste of a woman's beautiful energy.

Personally, I *rarely* weigh myself. My husband sometimes likes to see how much weight he drops after our long hikes and he'll ask me if I've weighed in. "No," I always say. I just hiked 115 miles and I feel great! A number is irrelevant. Do I feel energized? Is my skin glowing? Is my yoga practice progressing? Can I carry forty pounds on my back for twenty miles? Can I carry my five-year-old up the stairs when he falls asleep in my car? Do I feel sexy? If the answer is less than a resounding "yes!" I check in with my routine and get back on the Path. If my body is healthy and I'm happy, why would I care about numbers like weight and age? I don't let them preoccupy my mind or determine my self-esteem.

I happen to weigh a lot for my height. No one ever believes me when I tell them how much I weigh. At times, doctors have told me at annual physicals that I should keep an eye on my weight. If that doesn't make you preoccupied with a meaningless number, I don't know what will. And for years I was! I hated feeling that way. I reject the whole concept. What matters is how much muscle you have, how dense your bones are, how much body fat you have, not to mention how strong and energized you feel. So when my patients lament that they "feel fat," or that "if I could just get to [insert number here] pounds, I would be happy," I ask them to stop weighing themselves daily, find a positive marker for body happiness, and say, "I want to feel healthy/strong/fit/vital/energized/like a badass Goddess!" Don't obsess with the scale. Take joy in moving up your mountain toward homeostasis, one step at a time.

So, no, fat is not a feeling and, yes, pounds are just numbers. But "healthy" is a feeling, the best one you can have.

Hunger is also a feeling. Recognizing it will be one of the most important and valuable tools you'll integrate into your life during the eight weeks on the Well Path. You'll learn to see hunger as a positive, a sign your body is working as it should. You'll stop associating it with negative emotions. Even more important, you'll stop responding to uncomfortable feelings by eating.

You are undoubtedly familiar with what is known as emotional or stress eating. The phrase itself works in more ways than you think. Many women can relate to responding to stress, difficult emotions, or just feeling crappy with food, especially high-fat, high-sugar goodies. A sad woman eating ice cream is a cliché for a reason. I remember when I was a medical resident, pulling twenty-four-hour shifts, and I was bone-tired, even after working the obstetrics shift, which I loved. After an all-nighter, God help you if you were standing between me and a box of cookies. I was a mad cookie eater. The sugar and fat—and corresponding hit of feel-good hormones in my brain—alleviated the crappy sensation of sleep deprivation. It's been well documented that eating junk food in response to stress is addicting, just like a drug. In fact, researchers from the University of New South Wales in Sydney, Australia, have proven that going cold turkey on junk food causes a kind of withdrawal, which perpetuates the vicious cycle, causing more stress.

Cookies were my drug. To this day, when I'm sleep deprived or otherwise uncomfortable, I get "hungry" for cookies. It's been twenty years since my residency, and those neural pathways to my brain's reward center are still present. But now, having been in homeostasis for many years, I'm aware of my body's internal conversation and can distinguish false hunger from real hunger. That insight enables me to resist the cookie. I know that I'm not really hungry. I'm just uncomfortable—and I have better strategies to deal with that.

I don't need to tell you that certain times of the day make you more susceptible to stress eating, because you live this reality every day. But now science has proven that some hours are more witching than others. A study published in 2015 in the journal *Appetite* described an experiment in which researchers tracked the stress-hunger response in forty-five subjects, mostly female, over the course of a week. They found that the subjects tended to stress eat on weekday evenings, and in the later afternoon on weekends. My patients have told me over the years that their willpower peters out as the day goes on. They just get tired of being "good." By evening, they just don't have the *oomph* to fight it. I will reiterate here that you cannot will yourself to not eat. When you try to be "good" all day, exhausting yourself by ignoring pangs and being obsessed with intake, *of course* you'll be nuts for food come early afternoon and evening when all of your bodily systems are screaming and your real hunger is entangled with a half dozen uncomfortable sensations.

Eating for any reason but physical hunger puts your body at war with itself. Every forkful becomes loaded with emotion and hormonal mayhem. Food can and should be a source of pleasure and fuel for life.

What Are You Hungry For?

When I discuss hunger with patients, they can go into exhaustive detail about their eating plans and snack choices, how diets that promise to curb their appetites make them obsess about food—especially food they're not "allowed" to eat. I listen, and then I ask, "What are you really hungry for?"

They ask me what I mean.

"What do you *like* to eat?" I ask.

Still, they don't tell me what they *like* to eat. They tell me what they *do* eat. There is a difference. No one really likes eating plain egg whites for breakfast. How can anyone expect their body to be satisfied and refueled after eight hours of overnight fasting with seventy-five calories of tasteless egg whites? Will that tiny bit of nutrition power you through a morning of getting the kids to school, walking the dog, negotiating the commute, working, and running errands? No wonder you feel plagued by hunger. Your body loves you, and it's sending you a message to love it back. Give it some egg yolk!

Hunger, on an emotional level, is a metaphor for fulfillment. Satisfaction and satiety are the same thing. For those who struggle with weight, the connection between emotion and hunger feels like carrying a heavy backpack that's too big to bear even the smallest distance, much less up the mountain of fat loss. By understanding your deeper needs (such as love, friendship, fulfillment, security, acknowledgment, power, connection), you can gain a better understanding of how eating, our first form of fulfillment and pleasure, becomes a replacement for what we really hunger for in our lives.

Whatever that may be, it's not on the menu at McDonald's or in a pint of ice cream. Nor can it be addressed and changed overnight. If you can begin to break the subconscious connection between one type of hunger and another, you will feel an enormous sense of agency and relief. This work doesn't have to be emotional; it only requires a lot of patience, kindness, and honesty. I promise that the Well Path won't force you through deep self-analysis to work out your emotional connection with food and where it comes from. But I will give you the tools to distinguish real hunger from emotional hunger, and that having this awareness will significantly lighten your backpack. It's okay to leave the heavy stuff behind for now and just move forward. When you are ready to go back for the deeper psychology, your body will be in homeostasis and you'll feel stronger to face what you need to face. Or maybe you will just naturally let it go. The Well Path is focused on making strides to improve your well-being. Sometimes, those strides start with baby steps. Every inch forward is progress.

"I can't tell when I'm actually hungry or full."

Some of my patients have been dieting since their teens. They haven't experienced a healthy hunger feedback loop their entire adult lives. I had a long talk with one woman about her problem of not knowing the difference between real and false hunger. She was obsessed with the idea that she'd stretched out her stomach due to so many bingeing episodes, and that now she had to overeat to feel full. The stretched stomach is a myth. Your stomach will expand to accommodate a lot of food, but it snaps right back to normal size after digestion (and unless you're a professional athlete or have a rare metabolic disorder, it's unlikely that you digest a full meal in less than a few hours, anyway).

In my patient's case, we discovered that she would eat whenever she felt the slightest pang, making the tiniest bit of hunger intolerable. She was also eating nutrient-poor food. The combination of these behaviors was causing her hunger response system to send mixed or inaccurate signals. I asked her to run through the Hunger Checklist every time she felt a pang. By doing this multiple times a day, sometimes dozens of times, she was able to discern the difference between real and false hunger. And when she was hungry, she fueled her body with nutritious food, allowing her to feel full and satisfied. Eventually, she let go of her belief in a "stretched-out stomach" and no longer felt compelled to overeat.

The Hunger Checklist

When you feel a pang, don't immediately react by eating. First, triage the hunger to determine if it's real or false by running through the following eight-question list.

☐ When did you last eat? If you ate less than three hours ago, you may not be truly hungry. It takes that long for the food to move from the stomach into the small intestine.

☐ Did you eat enough at your last meal? You can fill your stomach with the volume equivalent of a baseball: a sandwich, a salad, a bowl of soup (go soup!), a piece of fruit, half a Chipotle burrito. If you ate an adequate volume of food, then you are probably not really hungry.

☐ Did you eat nutritionally dense food? Nutritionally poor food is not going to sustain you. Was your last meal a baseball-size serving of sweet dough? Starch and sugar are notorious for racing through your digestive system without supplying nutrients for cells, leaving you just as hungry as you were before you ate them, hence the phrase "empty calories." On the other side of the plate, nutrient-dense, high-fiber calories are "full calories."

☐ Are you thirsty? So often, hunger is mistaken for thirst. Have a big glass of water, hot tea, or hot lemon water.

☐ Are you eating out of habit? The body anticipates being fed. If you usually have a snack at 3 p.m., you'll be hungry for it, even if you had a late lunch.

☐ Are you uncomfortable? Search your feelings, physical and emotional. What are you experiencing? Is it stress, fatigue, sadness, anger, fear? Eating is a short-term solution to feeling uncomfortable.

☐ Is food right in front of you? Our society's access to food has evolved light-years ahead of our genetics. Our feast-or-famine mechanisms were not built for a twenty-four-hour drive-thru, or even a refrigerator. When our ancestors saw food, they ate it because they didn't know when or where their next meal was coming from. So we still have the impulse to eat everything we see on a buffet line, in a candy bowl, on a coworker's desk, or just driving past a Starbucks—even when we know it's not good for us.

☐ Are you bored? Boredom is an uncomfortable feeling. Eating is pleasurable. So if you've got nothing to do, it's only natural to think, "Let's get something to eat." People eat while waiting at the airport for their flight, watching TV, or at a boring event or lackluster party. Food is there when nothing else is. Hunger has nothing to do with it.

If you've gone through all the questions and are still convinced that your stomach is good and truly empty, then by all means *eat*! If you don't satisfy your hunger, you can't hope to right your hormones, feed your cells, and achieve homeostasis.

Reset Your Hunger Point

When they initially come in to see me, most patients describe having hypersensitive, reactionary hunger impulses. They're "hungry all the time." When they feel the slightest pang, they panic.

On the Well Path, you won't ignore your hunger, but you also won't eat every time thoughts of food enter your mind. Instead, you'll learn to be mindful of your hunger and experience it as a physical sensation like a sneeze or a tickle. In order to reset your hunger point, you have to understand it, and yourself. As I've said, when one system is off, the others are off, too. An out-of-control appetite is a neon-flashing sign that other areas of your health are in trouble. When you hit the reset button on your hunger, you'll be better able to heal the rest of your body as well.

The hunger reset strategies that follow might feel odd or uncomfortable at first. But if you follow the Path, hunger won't seem like an enemy anymore. It's not a friend, either. It is just a basic human function.

Hunger Reset Button #1: Get some sleep!

Insomnia can boost ghrelin production by 28 percent, and muffle leptin by 18 percent. One of my first questions for new patients who want to lose weight is, "How are you sleeping?" You can't reset hunger unless you're getting adequate rest. (Turn to page 156 for sleep strategies.)

Hunger Reset Button #2: Feel it, don't feed it.

We all have a set point for hunger, when we feel like we *must* eat. It's set pretty low, a holdover from our ancestors who were hungry all the time. To reset your hunger set point, try my mantra, "Feel it, don't feed it." Your ability to feel hunger and not immediately feed it is like a muscle that can be strengthened. Taking a moment between feeling and reacting allows you to practice awareness of the hunger type. I compare it to potty training a toddler. At first, they rush to the bathroom when they get the urge. Over time, they slow it down and don't react immediately. They train themselves to hold the sensation longer and longer. Their reaction time "muscle" gets stronger and stronger. Eventually, they can wait until an appropriate time and place to relieve themselves.

While your hunger "muscle" is developing, you'll become more mindful of your urges. You can feel a twinge of needing to pee, and comfortably sit with it, knowing it's there without panicking or suffering, and going to the bathroom when convenient or absolutely necessary. The point isn't to burst your bladder or starve yourself, but to slowly, consciously, train your hunger set point to shift to adapt to modern life and to give you the space to step back and assess where your hunger is coming from.

Hunger Reset Button #3: When you feel it, see it.

Visualization is a way to think about hunger before you respond to it. Picture hunger in your mind. I see it as an airplane. It flies into my peripheral vision, taxiing to the front of my mind, sitting for a minute before moving out of my airspace. When I see it, I acknowledge it and, with emotional detachment, run through the Hunger Checklist. Is it real hunger, or false? Do I really need nutrition, or is it something else? Visualization gives you the opportunity to discern if the hunger is real, a sensation like a tickle, or an itch or a sneeze, telling you that you need *fuel*. You don't fill up your car with gas when you're angry, frustrated, sad, bored, tired, or anxious. Why fill up your body when you feel that way? When those uncomfortable feelings are present, you should probably just send that hunger-pang plane into a holding pattern.

Hunger Reset Button #4: When you feed it, feed it well.

You can't eat a fat-free yogurt for breakfast and expect all systems to be "go." A healthy and nutritious diet doesn't mean tasteless or unsatisfying. It means a full variety of whole foods that provide a cornucopia of nutrients eaten throughout the day. You would never "water down" the gasoline you put in your car. I won't ask you to give up your favorite foods, but I will help you *nutrify* them. Eventually, eating like this will awaken your natural instinct to fuel your body in an optimal way. You'll gravitate toward the healthful combinations on your own.

To "feed it well," eat foods that have the most nutrient bang for the calories. I call that "nutrient-dense" food. You'll find whole foods the most filling. In 1995, a team of researchers from the University of Sydney in Australia compiled a list called "A Satiety Index of Common Foods." They compared subjects' feelings of fullness after eating 240-calorie portions of thirty different foods. Their findings were subjective, based on the personal opinions of the eaters. I find it to be spot-on. Heavy food by weight, like fruit and root vegetables, kept subjects satisfied for longer periods, as did high-protein food (beans, fish, eggs, and beef) and high-fiber food (fruit, lentils, oatmeal, bran, and popcorn). Whole foods performed best. Refined complex carbs like rice, bread, and cereal landed in the middle. The absolute worst choices were, not surprisingly, sugary foods and highly processed junk. Not only will whole foods give you more nutrients, they'll satisfy your hunger, keeping you full longer.

Dear Hunger Diary, I'm Freaking STARVING!!

Many diet plans advise followers to keep a food journal that allows them to track and then tally up all of the calories they've consumed each day. The problem with this practice is not only that it's tedious, but also that most food diarists tend to lie, or shave the numbers. When you lie to yourself in this way, it erodes the soul—not a good strategy for wellness. I don't advocate keeping a food diary because counting calories is counterproductive. It makes people obsessed with food, and provokes negative emotions like guilt and anxiety. Anything that makes someone feel bad is bad for weight loss, bad for self-esteem, and not found on the Well Path. I am an advocate of recorded assessment, though. But instead of a food journal, you will keep a Hunger Diary.

The Hunger Diary is an uncomplicated chart that is intended to help you notice your eating patterns. Do you typically get hungry around the same times each day? What do you usually eat? When do you usually eat? What were you feeling? As you track your relationship with hunger over time, you'll begin to shift your focus to "feeling, not feeding," thereby increasing your awareness to the needs of your body. You'll also use visualization techniques to assess hunger intensity and type. Before long, you'll know why you feel hunger and how to respond appropriately. After one month on the Path, your hunger hormones will be in balance and your hunger point will be reset.

8.

Activity

Humans are not designed for a sedentary, indoor lifestyle. We're supposed to be active from the moment we wake up until we go to sleep. By "active," I mean just moving around—walking, cooking, chasing children, dusting the cave. Our ancestors didn't take cars or trains to work, or drive the kids around. They didn't use modern conveniences. Everything was done by hand with physical effort. If they needed to get somewhere, they walked. When you're constantly at "rest," your body assumes that you need to conserve energy to gear up for the next round of hunting and gathering. Consistent activity with occasional bursts of exercise, followed by adequate rest, is the movement pattern our bodies were designed for. Our digestive, endocrine, and circulatory systems respond beautifully to it.

But, of course, that's not how we live now. Our pattern is more like low to no activity for long periods of time, followed by short, inconsistent bursts of exercise and inadequate rest. Our digestive, endocrine, and circulatory systems have been dismantled by it.

The unprecedented level of inactivity in our culture is fast destroying our health. When my patients fill out an Inactivity Chart—just a tally of how many hours they are on their butts during the day—they're shocked at how sedentary they actually are. We've basically stopped moving throughout our day, and it is literally killing us. The shift is both subtle and dramatic. Once upon a time, we got up from our desks to have a conversation with a colleague. Now, we text or e-mail. Once, we got up and had lunch outside the office. Now, we eat at our desk to eke out one more hour of work. We used to prepare our meals, standing up in the kitchen. Now, we order in. We used to shop on our feet, pushing a cart. Now, we click a button. You might think that driving to the mall to try on clothes doesn't burn many calories, so what's the difference, especially if you hit the treadmill three times a week? Well, when you add up all those hours of inactivity, a few hours at the gym don't make a dent. Inactivity perpetuates inactivity. Sitting for prolonged periods throughout the day actually makes you tired. It creates a vicious cycle of fatigue, exercise avoidance, excess calorie consumption, and slowed metabolism, not to mention feeling like crap, which then keeps the cycle going.

Activity heats the body, hence the medical phrase "non-exercise aerobic thermogenesis," or NEAT. Thermogenesis means "expending energy." NEAT is the energy that we expend, the calories we burn, doing everything except sleeping, eating, and exercising. NEAT has a cumulative effect on overall metabolism. For most people, NEAT is a more powerful contributor to your BMR than exercise, both in the total number of calories you burn and in priming the body to burn calories during exercise more effectively. Activity gets your circulation moving, bringing the good stuff in and moving the bad stuff out. It readily mobilizes liberated fat.

I want to be clear that activity is *not* exercise. Exercise is when you sweat and raise core body temperature. Exercise is what you do to become more fit. It's necessary and vital for strength and health. Hitting the treadmill for a few hours a week is not adequate compensation for sitting all day. However, if you exchange an hour of sitting for an hour of activity, you get a two-hour swing in the right direction for metabolic benefit every day. Two for the price of one. Who doesn't love that?

One additional hour of movement a day might seem like a lot, given how busy you are. But if you integrate it in a systematic way, starting with just 15 minutes a day, it's quite easy to work in. I'll show you how to do it on the Path. It will soon become second nature and you will be on your way to burning up to 400 extra calories a day, improving your circulation, and priming your body for improved fat metabolism during exercise without thinking twice about it.

The second magical benefit of NEAT is that it makes your exercise efforts even more effective. If you're moving around throughout the day, your body is primed to burn more fat when you engage in strenuous physical activity. According to a 2012 article in *Physiological Reviews*, subjects who engaged in "low-level activity" during the first half of the day amplified their lipolytic response—the process by which, as you'll remember, the fat cells leak FFAs—during their afternoon or evening workouts.

My favorite non-exercise activities are gardening, walking, and preparing soup (yay, soup, again!). I rarely get to garden, but when I do, I can spend hours doing it because I love it. I walk everywhere I can in any weather. Yes, this California girl has learned to love walking to work through Central Park in a snowstorm. I walk two miles through the park in the morning to my office, and two miles back as part of my daily commute. When I talk about my NEAT day to patients, they often say, "I'll get sweaty" or "I don't have the right shoes" or "I don't want to have to change when I get to work." Ladies, these are excuses. Logistics can be figured out if you put your mind to it. And remember, non-exercise activity is defined by not sweating. If you get too hot, slow down.

Fifteen minutes is just 1 percent of your day. Obviously, the more active you are, the bigger the bang for your buck. Once you start with those 15 minutes, you'll find that being more active will come naturally; being active perpetuates being active. It's basic physics. The difference in how your body feels on being NEAT versus being sedentary is profound. Not sitting for prolonged periods will change your life. On the Well Path, you only need to take one step at a time to get to your NEAT goal.

Being sedentary is more than just hazardous to your waistline—it can be deadly. Researchers have linked sitting for long periods of time with obesity and metabolic syndrome—a cluster of conditions that includes high blood pressure, high blood sugar, high cholesterol, and excess belly fat. Too much sitting also increases your risk of death from cardiovascular disease and cancer. One recent study by researchers at University College London compared adults who spent less than two hours a day sitting in front of TVs or computers versus those who logged four hours. The four-hour group had a 50 percent increased risk of death from any cause and a 125 percent increased risk of cardiovascular disease. An hour of exercise at the gym, even daily, doesn't offset the increased risk of sitting so much. Gym rats can also be couch potatoes, and their internal inflammation markers can be just as high as those who don't exercise at all. The researchers concluded that you have to be more active *throughout* the day during desk and leisure time to ward off these diseases and the higher risk of others, not to mention weight gain, rapid aging, and cellulite (gasp!).

Fifteen Non-Exercise Activity Ideas

Balance. While you're waiting in line to check out at the store, do a modified tree pose. Stand on one foot and place the sole of the other against your calf muscle. Square your hips, engage your core muscles, and breathe deeply while balancing. Don't forget to switch sides. In five minutes, you'll double the calorie burn of just standing.

Cook dinner rather than ordering in. It's not so easy! You have to stand to chop and stir, and bend to look in the oven, lift the casserole to the counter, and do the dishes afterward. Every micromovement is another handful of calories you wouldn't burn by ordering your dinner online. Goes without saying, home cooking is *always* healthier than takeout, so it's a win-win.

Dance. Put on music while cooking, cleaning, and commuting. Even slow jams can burn extra calories.

Exit. If you commute daily via public transportation, get off one stop earlier from the bus, tram, or subway. It adds only a few minutes to your commute, but you'll log activity before you get to work. This just requires preparation, and I will help you identify and carve out this time.

Fidget. Slim people tend to be fidgety. Even sitting, they're in constant motion. All that wiggling can burn up to 300 calories a day. If you are a squirmer, don't be shy or try to stop it. Jiggle your leg, twiddle your thumbs. Twitch to your heart's content.

Laugh. Laughing is a balm for the heart and the soul. In a study published in the *International Journal of Obesity*, researchers showed study participants either a drama or a comedy. The subjects who watched the comedy and laughed had a measurable difference in heart rate and calorie burn than the subjects who watched the drama—20 percent higher, in fact. In fifteen minutes of laughing, you can burn forty calories and get a boost of metabolism-friendly growth hormone.

Lift. Carry groceries instead of using a cart. Rearrange a bookshelf. Tote the bags up and down the stairs. Do leg lifts when you're chained to your desk. Lift the kids over your head. They'll love it, and so will your muscles, heart, and metabolism.

Pace. Instead of just standing there while you wait for a train or a flight, pace. I recently paced the subway platform for seven minutes, and, according to my Jawbone fitness tracker, I covered half a mile and burned sixty calories. It was more entertaining to pace than to just stand there impatiently. I was glad to wait, reducing stress, upping happy hormones, and getting in some steps at the same time. Win-win-win.

Park a block farther away than you ordinarily would. Walking the equivalent of one city block will burn twenty calories and expose you to sunlight for a hit of mood-boosting vitamin D.

Play with your kids outside instead of on the computer. If you engage your kids off-screen, they, too, will benefit from extra physical activity (not to mention your undivided attention). You will not only burn extra calories, but also bond with your kids and lower your stress level.

Shop. Burn fifty calories in fifteen minutes browsing through a store and trying on a new dress. Save $60 in fifteen minutes by not buying it.

Stand. If you have an office, look into a standing desk. Sometimes it's as simple as getting an inexpensive elevated platform for your keyboard that allows you to type while standing. Stand at home, too—when you talk on the phone, watch TV, whenever you can. Standing burns twice as many calories as sitting. If you do have to sit for prolonged periods, get out of your chair and move around one minute per hour.

Stretch. Keep a yoga mat by your desk, and do a few stretches when you take a work break. Vinyasa, a three-step pose, takes less than one minute and burns five calories each cycle. Start in a downward-facing dog, go into a plank, bend your elbows to descend into a yoga pushup, keeping them close to your body, then extend your arms while arching your back into an upward-facing dog. Three in a row will invigorate circulation and rush blood to the brain to restore, wake you up, and fill your head with brilliant ideas.

Take the stairs. At work, climb the stairs to get from one floor of your building to another. At home, make yourself do chores that require you to climb up and down stairs a few times a day. When you're out and about, climb the steps inside of a store or shopping mall rather than take the elevator. Each flight of twelve steps nets you fifteen calories. If you're going up and down the stairs all day at work like me, those numbers add up.

Walk around the block, around the living room, to and from meals, and while running errands. Fifteen minutes of moderately paced walking burns fifty calories in fifteen minutes.

My medical center is on the third floor of a prewar building with no elevator. New patients remark about the difficulty of having to walk up two flights of stairs for their appointment. I tell them, "You're here to lose weight! Embrace any activity that's presented to you." The ladies always give me pained looks, like activity is yet another thing they have to work into their day. They're *tired*. They're under stress and pressure and they just want to lie down. I understand this urge to the marrow of my own tired bones.

I also know that feeling tired becomes your default *because* you're inactive. It's the same idea behind "I've tried everything and nothing works." Trying everything is why nothing works. Why do you feel too tired for activity? Because you're inactive. The *habit* of plunking down on the couch is the reason why you feel like you can't move at the end of the day, or throughout the day. It's the *only* reason. That goes for women who have injuries and health conditions. Unless you're dead, you can find some way to add movement to your life. Again, an inch forward is progress.

Being inactive is an active choice. When you sit down at your desk for four hours without getting up, you are choosing to cut off blood flow and lymph drainage to your butt. When you spread out on the couch for four hours at night, you are choosing to slow your metabolism to a crawl and start a chemical cascade that shortens telomeres and turns your insides to rust.

Now or never, break the habit of inactivity and feel so much better mentally, emotionally, and physically just by standing up and shaking off that rust. Make an active choice to be an active person. When you've changed your habits and ingrained the practice of getting up every hour and taking a short walk, you'll feel edgy and antsy if you don't do it.

A sick body is a body at rest. A healthy body is a body in motion. Which body do you want?

9

Nutrition

When patients arrive at my office for their first appointment and we begin to discuss their eating habits, they often say some version of the same thing: "I know what I'm supposed to eat. I read all the latest books and articles about food. I buy all of the right things. But it's not working!" Then we have a long chat, and I realize that their idea of a healthy diet is way, way off. They have to unlearn what they've believed for so long and start over from scratch.

I tell my patients that learning how to nutrify your body is like learning a new language. You would never expect to have a full conversation with a native speaker within a couple of weeks. You would start out by learning some basic words, then you would progress to putting the words into sentences. When you master that, only then can you have a conversation. So let's start out with some basic terms that you will need to know to make you fluent in good nutrition.

The QCE Metric

The word "diet" actually means "food and drink considered in terms of its quality, composition, and its effects on health." Most people misuse "diet" to mean reducing calories/carbs/whatever to lose weight. When you follow a D-word, you make changes on Day One that are too aggressive and too abrupt and that are nearly guaranteed to drive you crazy by Day Twenty.

I'm wary of any "diet" that tells you that you can't eat a certain food; I'm in love with a diet that assesses food based on the criteria of Quality, Composition, and Effect on health. This is what nutrition means on the Well Path. We will use this QCE Metric to help you create a diet that fuels your body in a nutritious, flavorful, satisfying way. If every meal or snack hits high marks on the QCE Metric, you are doing a great job.

The first step is Quality. Quality means the best you can afford. Quality in food, especially today with the prevalence of factory-farmed produce and meat, is extremely important. I won't get into the debate about the food industry in the United States, but buying the highest-quality food you can is crucial for your health, even if it costs a bit more (and it will). Don't drive yourself crazy with this stuff. Just ask yourself the following questions for quality control:

Is it fresh? Fresh means unprocessed, raw, whole, unfrozen, unheated, no added chemicals. FYI: "Fresh frozen" means fresh food that was frozen after it was harvested.

Is it organic? Organic means fruit and vegetables grown at a farm in soil without pesticides, fertilizers with synthetic ingredients, or sewage. Organic meat and dairy products are made from animals that aren't given steroids, antibiotics, or growth hormone. Look for the USDA-approved label on supermarket organic food.

Would you be proud to feed this to guests? Is this food something delicious, planned for and prepared with love and care that you know won't be harmful to anyone who eats it, including you?

The next step is Composition. Composition means variety and nutritional value. If your diet is composed of lots of fresh fruits, vegetables, nuts, seeds, legumes, ancient grains, and organic meats, great. If it's composed of "food products" made in factories with chemicals and additives, not great. The composition of broccoli or raw nuts is diverse, with lots of micronutrients, macronutrients, and fiber, and dense, with plenty of nutrient bang per calorie. The composition of a bag of chips made in a factory is limited, with hardly any nutrients per calorie (but plenty of chemicals and other junk you don't want). If you're not used to eating or creating meals out of whole foods, composition might take some getting used to.

These questions can help you decide whether a food passes the composition test:

Is the food whole? Whole food is recognizable as something that was once alive. On the nutritional label, the ingredient list is one item. "Ingredient: apples." "Ingredient: farro."

Is the food processed? Processed food started its life as one thing, say, corn, and was turned into something else in a factory, using heat and adding chemicals. How long is the ingredient list? Are the first few ingredients refined flour, sugar, salt, or trans fats? If so, it's processed. Even if it's organic, it's still a few steps away from whole. If you can't pronounce it, the likelihood of its being processed is high.

The third step is the Effect the food has on your health. Culturally, we've gotten so far away from real food that we have lost the connection between what we put into our mouths to satisfy hunger and what our bodies actually need. We don't eat enough nutrients and fiber. Our bodies are starved for them. To compensate, we eat huge quantities of high-calorie processed food that does nothing to supply us with what we need throughout the day. So we get hungrier, and eat more junk, and gain more weight, and so on.

Food should have the effect of satisfying your body's nutrient needs, giving you energy and getting you to homeostasis. The effect of your diet should be to make you look and feel vital. It should *not* have the effect of skyrocketing insulin, causing glycation, and slowing metabolism.

Use the following questions to assess a food's effect:

How will it affect my body? As you know, foods that are high in sugar, salt, trans fats, and chemicals will throw your body into chaos and set off a hormonal nightmare.

Will the food speed my metabolism and promote muscle growth? Whole, fresh, and organic grains, vegetables, fruit, and meat will feed your cells and increase fat metabolism. Processed, heated, and chemical-filled food will do the opposite.

Will it clean and purify my body fluids and tissues, or will it clog them with chemicals and toxins? Always read labels to see how many chemicals are in your food. If you consume the chemicals, they will get stuck in your lymphatic system, causing oxidative stress, which damages your cells; and they will occupy your liver, which could be otherwise engaged protecting your body and metabolizing fat.

"What if I want to eat something with no nutritional value, just because?"

Eat it! Some foods you eat will have no value below the neck. But if you make a hard and fast rule that you can't eat it, you will rebel. Don't deny yourself a bite or two of any food. Just call a spade a spade, or a croissant a croissant. Admit out loud that you are eating something you know won't do you any good—not to shame yourself, but to acknowledge the intent behind your eating and to be mindful about it. Many aspects of the Well Path are about mindfulness and awareness. By being honest with yourself, you remove the shame and guilt, while consciously gravitating toward healthier choices.

It's not hard to figure out where something falls on the QCE Metric. An apple and a bag of pretzels have roughly the same number of calories. The apple grew on a tree and looks the same from farm to table. It contains fiber, vitamin C, and potassium. The pretzels were made in a factory. They have few vitamins or minerals, but plenty of refined carbs and salt. An apple provides cell-nourishing vitamins and protein for repair and regeneration. A pretzel sets off a nightmare hormonal cascade that turns your insides into goo-clogged rust. Which is higher on the QCE Metric?

To Count or Not to Count?

I have never seen obsessive calorie counting succeed as a strategy for sustainable weight loss. That said, I do know that having a basic understanding of the quantity of calories of the foods you like is important. You have to undo years of disconnected eating. Having a ballpark idea of portion size and calories will help you be mindful about true hunger and overeating, even when it comes to quality ingredients. When your body is in homeostasis, you'll be more connected to your appetite and will be able to eat when hungry and stop when full, making calorie counting irrelevant. For so many of my patients, gaining this ability is empowering. What a joy it is to finally feel a basic and beautiful connection to the glorious machine that we live in!

Composition Class: The Four F's

In medicine, compliance is a huge deal. If you can't get someone to follow through on their physician's advice, even the best "program" will fail. As doctors, we learn to work with what's realistic for our patients. A successful, sustainable plan has to acknowledge that we are different, and that one size does not fit all. I could have ten women come into my practice all wanting to lose twenty pounds, and each one of them would leave with different eating recommendations. You can't tell a woman who's grown up eating bacon that she has to give it up forever. In fact, the second you tell her that, she will probably just go eat a bacon-wrapped bacon burger with a side of bacon. That's nature. The Well Path has been carefully designed to be flexible enough to accommodate your individuality so that you can sustain success for the rest of your life. What works for all women is making an effort to nutrify the composition of every meal.

My "composition class" is all about the Four F's of nutrition: fruit, fat, fiber, and fuel. Add them to every meal, and your favorite meals will help you, not hurt you.

Fruit. Fruit is one of nature's gifts. It's the perfect source of glucose, a substance you need to grow and rebuild muscles and to feed your carb-loving brain. All varieties of fruit are full of antioxidants that help sweep away accumulated oxidation rust and reduce inflammation that can cause diseases. Fruit also tastes great and has plenty of fiber. The darker the berry, or the more intense the color, the more nutrients it has to offer. Eat little bits of fruit, ideally locally grown and seasonal, through-out the day to replenish your body with its cornucopia of nutrients.

Fat. There's been a lot of controversy surrounding fat over the past decade. Butter is the bad guy—or is it? Olive oil's a hero, but coconut oil's better? It is hard to keep up with the information on fat. Let's start with something concrete: Eating fat does not make you fat. Fat is crucial for your cells to function optimally. Your body can't thrive without it. It is important to eat some fat at every meal.

Now, some fats *are* bad for you. Trans fats found in red meat, cheese, ice cream, margarine, and processed foods such as cookies and crackers raise LDL, aka bad cholesterol, the stuff that forms plaque in your arteries and leads to heart disease, and decrease HDL, aka good cholesterol, the stuff that chips away at the plaque to clear your vessels. Since you are going to shift away from processed foods to whole foods, your trans fat intake will shrink.

Other fats support your health, such as essential fatty acids (EFAs). Your body can't make these fats on it own, but it needs them to survive. Omega-3s and omega-6s are the key EFAs. On the Well Path, you'll eat plenty of foods that contain these types of fat. It's important to balance your omega-3s with your omega-6s, though. Americans tend to eat a preponderance of omega-6s (corn oil, potatoes, poultry, grains), so I've created Well Path recipes to add omega-3s (nuts, vegetables, fish, legumes) to your diet. Consuming balanced EFAs decreases your risk for heart disease, lowers cholesterol, and improves metabolism, cognitive function, and digestion. When I balanced my EFAs years ago, the first thing I noticed was an improvement in my skin. When you are healthy on the inside, you will glow on the outside.

EFA Foods

Dark leafy greens: kale, parsley, watercress, spinach

Fatty fish: salmon, sardines, trout, halibut, mackerel, tuna

Nuts: almonds, walnuts, cashews, peanuts

Oils: olive, canola, coconut, walnut

Seeds: flax, chia, pumpkin, hemp, sunflower

Shellfish: oysters, shrimp

Fiber. Remember back in the '70s, when Americans were skinny and no one seemed to have cellulite? The health craze back then was bran, aka plant fiber. Plant fiber is nature's intestinal scrub brush. It cleans your intestines of sludge that prevents your gut from absorbing nutrients to pass along to cells. Fiber slows down your digestion, giving you more time to absorb nutrients. In essence, it makes you feel fuller longer by balancing hunger hormones.

The average American's fiber intake is about half of what it should be. We should eat 25 to 30 grams per day; most Americans eat half, or 15 grams. Our diet is high in meat and processed food, both of which contain little fiber. Grains have gotten a bad reputation because of gluten and carbs; vegetables are too often relegated to a small corner of the plate. I advise adding diverse types of fiber to your meals so that your body gets it from as many sources as possible.

For optimal health, you should incorporate both soluble- and insoluble-fiber foods into your diet. What's the difference? Soluble-fiber foods dissolve in water in the intestines and are digested slowly for maximum absorption. Insoluble-fiber foods do not dissolve in intestinal water. They speed up bowel movement, prevent constipation, and ultimately lower the risk of heart disease. They also promote the growth of good bacteria in your gut. Our modern American diet, with a predominance of calories from animal sources, such as meat and dairy, and processed food, causes an overgrowth of harmful bacteria and a depletion of healthy bacteria in our guts, which, in turn, causes intestinal disorders and skin problems like eczema and rosacea. On the other hand, a proper balance of bacteria in your intestinal system is directly linked to weight loss and maintenance.

Trillions of microbes live inside your gut. Studies have found that, in lean people, the microbe population is diverse, including those that are good at breaking down high-fiber foods. Obese people have a much less diverse gut community. The question "Which came first: the limited intestinal microbial ecosystem or the obesity?" is a hot topic in the scientific world. The answer isn't cut-and-dried, nor does it really matter to those who want to populate their gut with good bacteria. Rest assured that you can increase healthy flora by eating high-fiber goodies, such as artichokes, leeks, broccoli, asparagus, beans, onions, watermelon, pears, bananas, and raspberries.

An increase of only 10 grams of fiber per day will help you to feel fuller and will prevent hunger pangs. A high-fiber diet has also been shown to help stimulate fat metabolism. A study conducted at SUNY Stony Brook linked a high-fiber diet to decreased insulin response. With less insulin circulating in your system, your body is more able to access stored fat for fuel, instead of tapping into your muscles for energy.

Fiber Foods

Soluble-fiber foods

> Berries: blueberries, blackberries, strawberries
> Grains: oatmeal, millet, farro, spelt
> Hard fruit: apples, pears
> Legumes: beans, lentils, peas
> Nuts: almonds, cashews, walnuts
> Seeds: popcorn, flax, chia, pumpkin

Insoluble-fiber foods

Grains: whole grain bread, quinoa, brown rice, couscous

Vegetables: carrots, celery, zucchini, broccoli, cauliflower, beets,
    Brussels sprouts, dark Swiss chard, kale, artichokes, sweet potatoes,
    russet potatoes

Fuel. By fuel, I mean protein. Okay, so protein starts with a P not an F. (Should we call it frotein?) Protein is the fuel your body needs to build muscle. Even though high-protein diets have been trending for the last decade or so, you still might not be getting enough quality protein if you are exercising to become more fit.

How much protein is enough? If you're strength-training regularly, you need about 1 to 1½ grams of protein per kilogram of body weight. Your body needs the amino acids in protein to build new muscle and to repair the muscle you're strengthening. A kilogram is equal to 2.2 pounds, so a 130-pound woman would benefit from eating 60 to 90 grams of protein a day. If your exercise is particularly intense, your protein needs would be in the upper range; if your exercise is moderate, you'd be on the low end. If you don't get adequate protein from food, your body will turn to internal sources to repair muscles—like the muscles themselves.

Just as there are essential fatty acids, there are nine essential amino acids that you must eat for optimal functioning. Provide your body with as wide a variety of plant- and animal-based proteins as possible. It's a misconception that you need animals for protein. You can actually get all of your essential proteins from a plant-based diet, if you prefer to eat that way. Along with the protein, you get a million other benefits from eating plants that you can't get from meat. Here are two quick examples:

- **Quinoa.** This ancient grain is a complete protein, meaning it has the nine amino acids you need to eat to live, and a few others, too—isoleucine, leucine, lysine, phenylalanine, tyrosine, cysteine, methionine, threonine, histidine, tryptophan, and valine. Throw in 8 grams of protein per serving, magnesium, iron, phosphorus, and plenty of fiber, and you've got a gluten-free superfood.

- **Brussels sprouts.** They are packed with eleven amino acids—tryptophan, threonine, isoleucine, leucine, lysine, methionine, cysteine, phenylalanine, valine, arginine, and histidine—as well as thiamin, riboflavin, iron, magnesium, phosphorus, vitamin A, vitamin C, vitamin K, vitamin B_6, folate, potassium, manganese, and 3 grams of protein per cup.

These are just two examples and look at how many nutrients each of them offers!

Powerful Plant Proteins

A lot of people think that meat is 100 percent protein. Not so! Per the USDA Nutrition Database, beef is 26 percent protein. Chicken is 25 percent. Eggs? Only 12 percent. You can get a better bang for your protein buck from many vegetable sources, which are also high in fiber and micronutrients. Here are a few:

Spinach—49 percent

Kale—45 percent

Broccoli—45 percent

Cauliflower—40 percent

Mushrooms—38 percent

Parsley—34 percent

Cucumbers—24 percent

Peanuts—24 percent

Green peppers—22 percent

Cabbage—22 percent

Almonds—21 percent

Sunflower seeds—21 percent

Tomatoes—18 percent

If you pitted 4 ounces of steak against 4 ounces of black beans, which do you think would be a better source of protein and other nutrients? Let's take a look and see how they stack up by the numbers:

4 oz Steak	vs.	4 oz Black Beans
24 g protein		24 g protein
17 g fat		0.6 g fat
320 calories		120 calories
102 mg high cholesterol		0 mg cholesterol
0 g fiber		9 g fiber

Have I convinced you yet? You just don't need to rely on animal protein to get the cellular building blocks you need to live long and healthfully.

How to Compose Balanced Meals

Now that you understand the Four F's, you can start to compose healthier meals from old standards. Start with a few meals you can easily master to build your confidence. Stick with the familiar at first. As you become more proficient in the kitchen, you can expand your repertoire. You'll make changes slowly, one step, one ingredient, one meal at a time.

I ask my patients to choose their three favorite breakfasts, three favorite dinners, and three favorite snacks. Then we put them through the QCE Metric and adjust the composition to make them as nutrient dense as possible. What fruit, fat, fiber, and protein can we add? Then we sit back and wait for the positive effects.

Nutrify for Energy

Gina, age thirty-five, came to me because she felt bloated and exhausted. She got winded just going up and down stairs, and thought she might be asthmatic. "I have this fat around my belly that wasn't there a few years ago, and I can't get rid of it," she said.

I diagnosed her as a Convenience Eater immediately. She had no idea how to cook and she ate every single meal out of a box she bought at the supermarket. I asked her, "What's your favorite breakfast?"

"Pancakes!" she said. Every day, she took frozen pancakes out of a box and put them in her toaster and doused them in corn syrup masquerading as maple. In terms of the QCE Metric, the frozen pancakes and fake syrup were a great big zero. I gave her a recipe for nutrient-dense pancakes. She tried making them and got good at it. The effect was immediate. She not only felt satisfied by making them fresh, she wasn't rushing to a vending machine for a morning snack at 10 a.m. anymore. By adding nutrients to her breakfast, she wound up eating fewer calories throughout the day. By the end of her eight-week Well Path, she lost ten pounds and eleven years from her metabolic age. The belly fat and wheezing? Gone. Since she completed the program, she's lost three more pounds and said, "I'm not even trying anymore. It's automatic."

Big Ideas about Food

Dieters tend to think really small about food. They count calories and grams, eliminate groups, limit choices, and obsess over tiny decisions. On the Well Path, I'll ask you to think bigger about food.

The first is to try to eat less dairy and meat. Ethical and Earth resource arguments aside, eating fewer animal calories is proven to contribute dramatically to disease prevention and weight loss. Meat and dairy are sludge in your digestive system, causing constipation, oxidation, and inflammation, which kills healthy enzymes and chokes cells. I'm not a big fan of diet labels. Vegan, vegetarian, carnivore, pescatarian, I don't care. The goal here is optimal health, and whatever choice you make as an individual should feel good to you. That said, I describe my own way of eating as a plant-based diet, or as my cousin Val says, "Flexitarian: She eats a plant-based diet, but is flexible on occasion." Eating mostly plants has served me well. Research suggests that the diet for optimal health would contain no more than 10 percent of daily calories from animals (meat, dairy, and eggs). That's about 200 animal-based calories per day, which may be a big shift to make all at once for many people. My advice is to just walk toward it, step by step, with a little less animal in each meal, each day, and then each week. You'll be surprised how little you miss it if the transition is progressive, and when you get the positive reinforcement of feeling better every step of the way.

The second big idea is to be mindful of how many steps it takes to produce the food. Corn is great if it is a non-GMO boiled or steamed ear, fresh and full of fiber. Corn chips that have been fried in oil or baked in a factory are chemical triangles held together with artificial colors and flavors, saturated fat, and AGEs. The fiber and vitamins have been replaced with chemicals, preservatives, and sodium. Instead of eating food with preservatives, eat pure to preserve your body. Strictly avoiding processed food altogether is another big leap for many, even myself. Ezekiel breads didn't come out of the ground packaged and sliced. Olive oil doesn't grow on trees already bottled. Just use common sense, and ask yourself, "How many steps from whole is this food?"

Another big idea: Forget labels on the box that make promises like "whole grain" and "natural." Any grain that comes in a box has been processed and stripped of nearly half its fiber. You may be better off eating the box.

How Food Labels Are Misleading

A label will try to sell you on a food's qualities, but don't be fooled by . . .

- "Whole grain." Unless it's 100 percent whole grain, it could contain just a tiny fraction of the good stuff.

- "All natural." Sugar is natural. Salt is natural. Corn syrup is natural. Some natural foods can be sky-high in sugar, fat, and salt. Check calorie and sodium content.

- "No sugar added." What about the sugar that's already in it? Or chemical sweeteners?

- "Sugar free." If something says "sugar free" and it's still sweet, you can assume that it's loaded with chemical sweeteners that have the same impact on your metabolism as real sugar.

- "Free range." This label would seem to mean that the beef or chicken or eggs in question originate from animals that are free to roam on a ranch. But it actually means they had exposure to the outdoors, possibly in a small cage with many other creatures. A "free-range" chicken can produce plenty of stress hormones and be fed a diet of grain instead of grass. "Cage free" is better than "free range." The best choices: cage free, grass fed, antibiotic free, humanely slaughtered.

- "Fat free." I always say to patients, "Fat free means sugar full and chemical full." If you take out the fat, you also take out the flavor. The manufacturer's solution? Add sweeteners and chemicals.

- "Light." Meaningless. This label can be put on food with 50 percent less fat than the un-light variety, but it can still be full of sugar and chemicals and have a ton of fat.

- "Gluten free." Take out the gluten and you have to put something in to give the food texture. If you want to avoid gluten, avoid bread and cake. If you buy "gluten-free" bread, choose Ezekiel products.

- "Made with real fruit." It might have a minuscule amount of fruit to meet the FDA requirement for the label. How about just eating real fruit instead?

- "Cholesterol free" and "Trans fat free." According to the FDA, these "frees" actually mean "a little." A cholesterol-free product can have 2 grams of cholesterol per serving. A trans-fat-free product can have half a gram of trans fat in it. Read the label for exact amounts. Or just choose naturally cholesterol- and trans-fat-free whole foods like fruits and veggies.

- "Organic." Just because a food is grown without chemicals doesn't mean it's not full of sugar and fat. "Organic" can be an empty promise when it comes to packaged food. Organic chocolate chip cookies are still chocolate chip cookies.

My last big idea on nutrition is to cook often and eat with people you love. Trust me, I know how hard it is to cook dinner on a busy weeknight. When I don't prepare ahead of time, I slip in that department. If you didn't hear my mantra the first ten times, here it is again: Just do the best you can! That's good enough.

Food you prepare yourself will always (*always*) be healthier and less expensive than what you'd get from a store or in a restaurant. Prepared or frozen foods from the supermarket contain chemicals and preservatives that wreak havoc on all of your delicate bodily systems. When you eat in a restaurant, you have no idea what ingredients are used in the restaurant kitchen. The cook doesn't care about the calories in the oil he brushed on your chicken to make it glisten. In your own kitchen, you have control. Also, cooking adds thermogenic activity to your day!

Build a menu of nutrified foods that you like, starting very simply and moving to more complex meals as you go along. Usually, I double or triple my recipes to freeze for when I have to work late or I'm simply not as prepared as I'd like to be. Cooking at home is also a huge opportunity to plant the seeds of good nutrition and healthy cooking skills in the minds of your children, so they learn to walk the Well Path sooner rather than later.

Gut Absorption

No matter what you eat, if your gut isn't absorbing nutrients properly, your cells won't get all the good stuff they need to thrive. As we get older, our gut—or our digestive tract—becomes less efficient at absorbing nutrients. Aging means that, paradoxically, our nutrient needs go up while our calorie needs go down. Hunger hormones kick into overdrive, but our gut is less able to absorb nutrients, causing us to overeat. That's one reason people tend to gain weight as they age.

When women turn sixty, they can expect to see a steep drop in healthy gut bacteria as well as an increase in less beneficial microbes. As a result, you're at higher risk for intestinal problems, from relatively minor woes like bloating and constipation to bigger ones like irritable bowel syndrome and colon cancer.

A healthy and diverse gut flora also boosts your immune system and helps to ward off inflammation, which is an underlying cause of heart disease, cancer, and diabetes. This is especially important as you age, since your immune system and healing ability are already compromised by a drop in stem cells. You need all the help you can get, and a balanced, thriving population of microbes will do you a world of good.

Here are a few of the strategies you will use on the path to improve digestive health:

Clean your colon. A gut check starts with eating more high-fiber fruits, veggies, legumes, nuts, seeds, and gluten-free grains.

Chew slowly. Chew until your food loses its texture. Thoroughly masticated food is absorbed by the gut; poorly chewed food is not. Picture spilling a glass of water on a towel. The towel soaks up the liquid easily. Now, throw a chunk of meat on the towel. It just sits there, correct? Well, readers, *the towel is your bowel.* I think women often eat quickly because they let themselves get so hungry that they scarf down their meals as if someone is going to snatch it right out of their hands. If you chew to liquefaction, you'll boost absorption and reset hunger hormones. In a week's time, you'll learn to eat like a rabbit instead of a wolf.

Colonize your colon. Eating fiber is key—it promotes the proper colonization of bacteria in your intestines—so eat plenty of veggies. Fermented foods like kimchi, sauerkraut, miso, kefir, kombucha, and yogurt contain naturally occurring probiotic cultures that help to maintain GI health. If you don't eat a lot of fermented foods, you might want to consider adding a probiotic supplement to your diet. I recommend the brand Enzymatic Therapy to my patients.

Irrigate it. A hydrated gut is a happy gut. You need fluid to keep things moving. If your digesting food is mixed with a lot of fluid, it's easier for your bowels to absorb nutrients. The rule of thumb is to drink half your body weight in ounces of water a day. That means a 150-pound woman should drink about seventy-five ounces of water a day, or two liters. If you live in a high-altitude or dry climate, add eight ounces to that. For every alcoholic beverage you drink, add another glass of water. Pregnant and breastfeeding women should also add a glass or two daily. How do you know if you're well hydrated? A good gauge is urinating about every two hours, and having clear urine.

Soup Is the Solution

According to a 2005 article in the *American Journal of Clinical Nutrition*, the modern American diet of processed foods is responsible for "diseases of civilization." Two-thirds of the U.S. adult population is affected by diet-related disease—like obesity, heart disease, diabetes, high blood pressure, and GI tract cancers. These conditions don't exist in hunter-gatherer societies, and are still rare in modern non-Western populations. Technology (tractors, refrigerators, GMOs, and chemical additives) has completely changed what we eat and how we eat, while our ancient digestive and metabolic systems have stayed the same. As a result, our population is becoming increasingly fat and sick.

Back in the caves, people threw whatever food they had into their version of a pot (a hollowed-out mammoth skull?), added water, and set it over a fire to cook. And it wasn't just our ancient ancestors who cooked this way—most of us grew up with grandmothers who were avid soup makers. The combination of animal bones and vegetables slow-cooked in water is the most basic way to preserve every nutritional drop of food.

Soup is also easy to digest, hydrating, packed with flavor, and super-satisfying. If homeostasis were a restaurant, every item on the menu would be soup.

I'm addicted to it. I cook soup every week, and spend whole days playing with ingredients and recipes. The recipes in this book are the result of years of study, experimentation, and research. When my husband and I hike the Appalachian Trail, going ten or twenty miles per day, we need lots of nutrients to keep us moving. I stuff my backpack with vacuum-packed bags of dehydrated soups to rehydrate on the trail over our little campfire. For days at a time, we eat *only* these soups and never feel hungry or deprived. We feel energized and strong.

A bowl of one of my soups will fill the holes of deficiencies in your diet and counteract the damage of classic Western eating. The recipes were designed, ingredient by ingredient, to supply your body with a harmonious balance of the nutrients you need to thrive.

Every recipe in this book is brimming with:

Fiber, protein, vitamins, and minerals. The American diet is low in more than a dozen vitamins and minerals, including vitamin A, vitamin B complex, vitamin C, magnesium, calcium, zinc, folate, riboflavin, thiamine, and phosphorus. A multivitamin isn't the answer. Not only does quality vary widely among brands, but your body doesn't absorb vitamins from a pill as well as it does from fresh, whole foods.

Phytosterols. These are compounds found in plant cell membranes (vegetable oils, whole grains, nuts, and legumes) and are close in structure to cholesterol. Our ancestors ate a ton of them. Modern humans?

Not so much. When eaten, phytosterols inhibit the absorption of cholesterol in your intestines, reducing your risk of Western-diet diseases while improving circulation and immune function and speeding metabolism.

Balanced essential fatty acids. My goal was to not only add omega-3 and omega-6 to the soups, but also to get the ratio of one to one as close as possible. Too much omega-6 can cause inflammation.

Balanced sodium–potassium ratio. Most of us are eating way too much salt—on average, 3,300 mg, or 1½ teaspoons, per day. We should consume 2,300 mg or less. Most of the salt we eat is made in a factory—which means it doesn't contain all of the naturally occurring and beneficial minerals found in sea salt. Only 13 percent of Americans eat the right amount of sodium.

We're also eating far too little potassium—2,600 mg. We should consume 4,700 mg, nearly twice as much. Only 5 percent of Americans get as much potassium in their diets as they need.

Too much sodium plus not enough potassium is a deadly combination. If the amounts are off, our body is out of pH balance and that interferes with intercellular communication, causing problems like migraines and muscle spasms. What's more, a diet that's high in sodium and low in potassium puts you at a significantly increased risk for hypertension, stroke, kidney stones, osteoporosis, asthma, insomnia, and GI tract cancers. However, if you get the ratio right—cutting sodium in half and doubling potassium—you can turn it all around and reduce your risk of these diseases.

All of the foods on the Well Path—fruits, veggies, whole grains, lean proteins—are low in sodium and high in potassium.

Herbs and spices. These secret anti-inflammatory weapons add flavor and contain phytochemicals and active compounds that boost overall health, hormone balance, and enzyme production. In the soups, you'll find tons of spices and herbs, including turmeric, oregano, cilantro, chili pepper, garlic, nutmeg, ginger, curry powder, cumin, paprika, thyme, cayenne, and rosemary.

Eat Your Soup!

I sound like your grandma, right? Eat your soup, bubala! Well, she was right. Soup is health and love in a bowl.

More than a dozen soup recipes start on page 249. Take a look. You'll see that soups are not complicated to prepare. No professional chef hat required. There might be an ingredient or two you haven't heard of before. Part of the Well Path is stepping ever so gently out of your old routines and into a brave new world that has chia seeds, hominy, and lemongrass in it. Every ingredient is available at most major supermarkets, definitely at Whole Foods, or can be ordered online.

10.

General Health

When I do intakes at my office, I try to get a sense of the patient's general health. I've found over the years that I can get an accurate sense of it just by looking at the quality of her skin, the brightness of her eyes, and by asking her questions about the Four S's: sleep, sex, stress management, and social interaction.

If a woman sleeps seven to nine hours per night, she gets a gold star on her chart.

If she has sexual activity and feels good about it at least twice a week—with a partner or by herself—she gets a happy face.

If she has a regular meditation practice, a spiritual or religious tradition, does yoga, is in therapy, or has some way to quiet her mind and connect with her soul on a daily or weekly basis, she gets a heart emoji.

If she describes herself as being involved in her community or in charitable causes, or she lives with people and has an active social life, she gets a big check mark.

These four categories, collectively and individually, play an enormous role in happiness, wellness, weight loss, and hormonal balance. You will need a solid baseline on all of them in order to be vital and youthful. As I've explained previously, all of our bodily functions are interconnected. That's why you can't just cut out sugar, for example, and expect to undergo a miracle whole-body cure. Your ultimate goal is the optimal functioning of total body homeostasis. It does take a little effort to get there. Just a little, though, and none of the Four S's will hurt. Who doesn't crave more sleep, more sex, sailing through the ups and downs of life, and connecting with and being helpful to others—preferably while getting large doses of nature? Sounds ideal to me.

Sleep

It's simply not possible to reach homeostasis without the restorative powers of adequate rest. Your body needs a minimum of seven hours of quality sleep per night. Unless you get that much, weight loss and restorative health are impossible. Yes, impossible. A dozen hormones that control appetite, metabolism, mood, and muscle growth are affected negatively by sleep deprivation.

A sleep-deprived body, like a food-deprived or stressed-out body, is in survival mode, keeping you alive until the famine, tiger attack, or earthquake is over. As we lie awake with insomnia, or pull an all-nighter to meet a deadline, our bodies perceive the stress and exhaustion as threats. The body doesn't know you have financial woes or a mean best friend. It only knows that you're not sleeping when you should be. Fat metabolism happens only when your body is relaxed and restored.

In 2012, researchers at the University of Chicago divided female study participants of similar weight into two groups. One group slept nearly eight hours per night for four nights. The other group slept four and a half hours per night. They ate the exact same meals. When the study ended and their fat cells were analyzed, the sleep-deprived subjects' insulin sensitivity *decreased* by 30 percent. The lead researcher concluded that sleep deprivation makes your fat cells "metabolically groggy."

Sleep, hunger, metabolism, and cell growth are intrinsically linked. I encourage all of my patients to get more sleep. Go to bed early. Take weekend naps! Tell your partner and kids, "I have to go lie down. I'm trying to lose fat and be healthier," and know you have science on your side.

There are just a few guidelines of good sleep hygiene that we should all uphold. To a one, the simple methods cured most sleep issues in a matter of weeks. In later chapters, I'll prescribe week-by-week goal setting, but for now, here's an overview:

Avoid caffeine after 2 p.m.

Exercise regularly, but not within two hours of bedtime.

Establish set sleep and wake times to reset circadian rhythms so your body knows when to feel tired and when to feel awake.

Take a one-hour buffer zone before bed when you relax *off-screen*.

Snack for Sleep

A sleep expert friend once told me that he encourages his patients to have a 100- to 200-calorie carb and protein snack an hour before bed. I have a snack every night before bed without fail. Pre-sleep snacking is a standard "diet" no-no. Well, on the Well Path, we don't care about D-words and their rules. The carbs bring a release of serotonin, the "happy" hormone, which helps people relax into sleep. The protein is filling and primes the body for muscle restoration while you rest. The hormonal benefit of sleep far exceeds an extra 200-calorie intake. You burn those calories the next day, when your appetite is well regulated and you have more energy for activity and exercise.

Some suggestions:

An apple or pear with almond butter

¼ cup hummus with a small handful of Mary's Gone Crackers

1 piece Ezekiel bread with 1 teaspoon nut butter and ½ teaspoon honey

¼ cup buckwheat groats, cooked with hemp or almond milk, chilled, and topped with ½ teaspoon honey or ¼ cup fresh or frozen fruit, 1 teaspoon chia or flax seeds, or 1 teaspoon crushed almonds, cashews, or walnuts

¼ cup warm steel-cut oats, cooked in hemp or almond milk, with
1 teaspoon nut butter and ¼ cup fresh or frozen fruit mixed in

¼ cup Ezekiel or Kashi cold cereal with hemp or almond milk,
topped with 1 teaspoon flax or chia seeds and 1 teaspoon
unsweetened coconut

Sex!!!

Sex is, hands down, my favorite wellness practice. And when I forget that it is, my husband reminds me of the importance of practicing what I preach. I can cite a thousand studies that show the benefits of frequent, satisfying sex: reduced risk of heart disease, pain relief, boosted immunity, improved circulation, better bladder control, healthier teeth, reduction of stress, anxiety, and depression, mental sharpness, and enhanced sense of smell (really). Humans evolved to seek out sex not only for the immediate purpose of procreation, but also to improve our health, therefore making us more attractive to potential mates and to keep us alive longer, lengthening our reproductive life span. The more orgasms you have, the healthier your body.

No surprise, hormones make the fun happen. A hormone called phenylethylamine (PEA) is released during sex, and offers a few bonus benefits: it's a fat metabolism stimulator and an appetite suppressant. Dehydroepiandrosterone (DHEA) comes into play when you're experiencing joy. A natural steroid, DHEA is produced by the same gland as cortisol (adrenal yin and yang) and is the hormonal equivalent of throwing logs on the metabolic fire. Since DHEA levels decline after age twenty, some experts think of it as a fountain of youth. It does, actually, stimulate growth of healthy skin cells. That glow you notice at the start of a new relationship when you're having tons of enthusiastic, aerobic sex? You can thank DHEA for that, along with a dozen other orgasm biochemical by-products like oxytocin and human growth hormone. A 2013 study conducted by British neuropsychologist David

Weeks tracked the sexual habits of thousands of subjects over a ten-year period. Researchers found that the middle-age subjects in their forties and fifties who had the most sex looked younger compared to their peers who had less frequent sex. Researchers suggested that the release of human growth hormone during intercourse may have been the cause for participants' youthful glow.

By the way, masturbation brings on the same hormonal cascade and is just as beneficial to your health as having sex with a partner. In a study of more than 2,500 women between the ages of twenty-three and ninety, 39 percent of the self-pleasurers in the bunch remarked on how relaxed they felt afterward. They can thank the post-orgasm release of soothing, calming oxytocin for that effect. When oxytocin level goes up, cortisol level goes down. Orgasm is your body's instant de-stress mechanism.

Orgasm benefits the brain, too. The amygdala—the brain's anxiety zone—becomes inactive when a woman has an orgasm. Orgasm has been shown to increase blood flow to every part of the brain, filling your smarts cells with nutrients and oxygen, and improving memory, concentration, and imagination. An orgasm is as mentally restorative as a nice nap. The Well Path is all about making mindful choices. Sexual activity, or any step leading toward it, is a better choice to make in the evening than watching TV and pigging out on the couch. Just saying.

Is Sex NEAT?

That depends on what kind of sex you like!

If you prefer it nice and slow, you can absolutely add sex to your list of non-exercise activities, burning about 100 calories per session. If you're more athletic in bed and raise your heart rate enough for sex to qualify as exercise, you can burn 200 calories per session and enjoy the metabolic afterburn along with your afterglow.

As a mother of three children ranging in age from five to sixteen, trust me when I say I know the mental hoops you have to jump through to get one more activity in at the end of a long day. Getting more sex into your routine can be a real challenge mentally, emotionally, and physically. There are many nights when curling up in bed and being left alone is the most appealing option—and, of course, it is absolutely okay to do that when you need sleep and alone time. For me, I know that once I push past the "I'm too tired" reflex, I appreciate just how contributive sex is to my mental and physical well-being. I'll reiterate my mantra that doing your best is good enough. Any step in a forward direction will put you ahead of where you are.

I have patients who haven't had sex with their husbands in years. "I don't miss it," one said recently. "It's just not a part of my life anymore." It's important for women to know that sex is the ultimate "use it or lose it" for us. Vaginal atrophy is a very real risk, especially for postmenopausal woman with nonexistent sex lives. After three years without sex, the opening of the vagina shrinks and eventually narrows so much that when you do try to have sex, it can be extremely painful. The condition of having pain during intercourse is called dyspareunia. If you ignore your sex life for an extended period now, it could seriously compromise your ability to enjoy sex a few years down the line. And there is a lot to look forward to: University of California researchers interviewed more than 800 postmenopausal women in a retirement community about their sex lives. Fifty percent of the women in the over-eighty category said their sexual satisfaction kept getting better with age, and that they experienced orgasms every time, or almost every time, they had intercourse. Don't miss out on all the fun you could be having when you make it to the retirement home!

Stress

I've already described what stress does to your health and appearance. It literally shows on your face. You might be totally stressed out about being stressed out. I used to hate it when people would tell me to "Just relax!" during stressful times in my life. Telling someone to relax when they're under intense pressure is not helpful. What can help is accepting, even embracing, that you are stressed out. In a recent Yale University study, researchers told half of their subjects that stress can be beneficial and not to worry about it, and instructed the other half that stress is debilitating and to be very afraid of it. In follow-up evaluations, the "beneficial" group reported significantly better psychological symptoms and work performance than the "debilitating" group. Merely telling yourself "Stress is good" helps to alleviate it. Sometimes, when I feel myself going down the rabbit hole, I say out loud, "Screw you, stress!" That does wonders.

Over time and with practice, I've learned to manage stress and discern which stressors to fight, which to flee from, and which ones not to react to at all. In the Well Path weekly planners, I'll guide you through a very specific exercise to triage your stressors, using a simple method to help you eliminate or counteract your responses to them. The strategies won't solve the problems or eliminate your stress, but they will train you to stop wasting precious energy reacting to stressors that are either inconsequential or that you have no control over.

Socializing

We all need to make more time for fun, friends, family, and community. This ranks as one of my top recommendations for people who are not enjoying optimal general health despite "doing all the right things." Socializing and/or volunteering gives us a sense of perspective and a feeling of gratitude. Volunteering is a term that I like to use to include any gift of kindness or generosity to another human being, not necessarily signing up at your local soup kitchen (soup!). Well-being naturally flourishes when you help others. My grandmother used to say, "When life gives you lemons, give lemonade to someone who's thirstier than you are." A growing body of research indicates that volunteering provides not just social benefits, but health benefits as well. Performing simple acts of kindness releases all the feel-good hormones that lift you up emotionally and physically and are necessary for finding internal balance.

And, in fact, the insta-cure for stress and anxiety just might be kindness. Researchers at the University of British Columbia asked their anxious subjects to perform random acts of kindness six times a day for four weeks. The worriers went about their regular lives as usual, but added various generous gestures to their days, like holding doors open for strangers, helping someone carry their groceries, donating goods, or treating friends to lunch. After four weeks, the subjects' anxiety was shown to have significantly diminished. They were also less shy, and sought out more mood-boosting social situations. I'll add that being kind doesn't cost a thing or require a prescription.

Making a habit of daily positive interaction, no matter how small, is a subtle mind shift, but one that is well worth making. Multiple studies have found that if you can find the time to volunteer or do charity work, your altruism and service to the community will be rewarded with a longer life, greater satisfaction, reduced depression, and better general health.

I always ask myself, Why are we here? What is the point of being alive? What gives us the most joy? Human beings are social creatures by design. What would life hold for us if we didn't work and live together? When we are isolated, we suffer. When we are together, we thrive. It's true for your weekend, and your physiology.

Social Drinking on the Well Path

Does being social have to include social drinking?

I'm not going to tell anyone not to drink a glass of wine at dinner once or twice a week. It's absolutely fine as long as you counterbalance it with plenty of water and nutritious food.

But . . . your liver can't do its job of processing fat if it has to first occupy itself with getting rid of toxins you put into your body, including alcohol. The liver is smart, and it has a priority list. Filtering out poison to keep you alive is number one. Getting rid of fat is further down on the list.

If you want to lose fat, reduce the toxins you introduce to your body. Drinking more than two glasses of wine, bottles of beer, or cocktails per week will sabotage your weight loss, especially in the beginning.

I can tell you that when women are on the Well Path, they often lose their taste for alcohol. They just don't want to drink. When your body is in balance, you crave what's good for it. The desire to drink diminishes or disappears completely. It's kind of shocking, actually. The same thing happens with tastes for junk and sugary food. It's quite natural for your body to want healthy food and not want alcohol when you reach homeostasis. Nothing tastes as good as homeostasis feels.

Of course, there is also an emotional component to this shift. Drinking is often a way to self-medicate, especially for busy women. When you are stressed and unable to cope, you reach for alcohol to make the sharp edges of your day a bit softer. On the Well Path, you'll learn to cope with stress in a healthier way, and you won't need to self-medicate.

11

Exercise

Get off the "dreadmill." Literally and figuratively.

For so many women, their idea of exercise is getting on a treadmill for thirty minutes or more. But I can assure you that these workouts won't get you where you want to go. They don't help your body to metabolize fat; they don't improve balance, flexibility, or upper body strength; and if you aren't really exerting yourself, they're not even strengthening your lower body muscles. In fact, the classic treadmill routine actually *slows* metabolism and *encourages* the body to hold on to fat. I'm not talking about serious athletes who train for hours a day and eat thousands of calories to maintain their muscle mass and energy level. I'm talking about regular women who hit the gym religiously three times a week, put in their time, hate it, force themselves through it, and still never lose weight. And yet they persist, because they believe they have to or all hell will break loose.

Working out is about so much more than burning calories on a treadmill or elliptical machine. Exercise should serve two purposes: fun and fitness. If you achieve these goals, your efforts will be worth the valuable time you invest and will make fitness sustainable for the rest of your life. Working out with the sole purpose of losing weight is a fool's errand. Life is about balance—for your body, your brain, and your spirit. If you put all of your energy into forced repetitive workouts that you loathe, you are sending your whole system into a tailspin. On the other hand, having a varied exercise routine that you find fun can help you to be active and strong for your whole life. That *is* what you really want, right? For your body to perform what you ask of it, whether you're playing with your kids or grandkids, hiking a mountain, snorkeling a reef, or just getting the day's chores done with youthful vigor, pain free. Skinny has nothing to do with performance. Physical capacity is a direct line to feeling like a badass Goddess. The fat will come off while you're having fun.

The first step on this exercise path is to shift your thoughts and goals from dread and failure to fun and success. I'm forty-seven, and I've cycled through the love/hate relationship that many women have with exercise. At this point in my life, if an exercise isn't fun for me, I don't do it. Growing up, I played sports. I loved being part of a team and working hard toward a common goal. In college I made the volleyball team, but eventually quit—I didn't enjoy *that* team experience—and wound up playing in doubles tournaments with a partner. Volleyball was fun again. Along with fitness, a powerful lesson took hold. Working that hard can't be sustained if you're not having fun and progressing toward a meaningful goal. Life is too short to hate what is supposed to make you feel happy.

Not to say that what once made you happy will now fit into your life perfectly. A friend of mine was a big runner in her twenties and into her thirties, but after thirty-five, it just stopped feeling good for her. She went through an exercise dry spell and gained weight because she dreaded lacing up her sneakers. On a lark, she tried spinning, fell in love, and got her exercise mojo back. My point is that exercise should feel fun for wherever you are in your life now. Not you in your twenties or you last week.

On the search for fun, you will try new things, and do them with friends and have fun, get fit, and love your body for what it will be able to do for you!

Fun

When I meet with new patients, I ask, "What type of exercise do you enjoy?"

Most answer, "I hate exercise."

Okay, next question. "What exercise have you enjoyed in the past, like when you were a kid?"

Almost always, a smile comes across their faces and they light up recalling some fun thing they used to do. That's the emotion I want to see. It's in your nature to have fun with exercise, to make it a game, like when you played tag or kickball when you were a child. You need to get back to a sense of joy and identify an exercise that feels like play. Everyone has those memories buried deep somewhere. If patients can't recall something, I ask, "What exercise have you never tried that seems like it would be fun?" Be it hang gliding or trapeze, surfing or horseback riding, without fail, we come up with a few options.

Not that they volunteer to rush into doing it. The prospect of trying a new exercise when you are not fit can produce palpable fear. Fear and lack of fun are why we get stuck in a rut. They perpetuate the cycle of failure. When I was forty-two with fifty pounds to lose, I couldn't even walk up the stairs to my office without gasping for breath. Every step was painful. I shared my fear and anxiety about the mountain ahead of me with one of my best friends, Lisa. She had just started spinning classes and told me I should go with her. Biking had been a favorite activity back in college. My first reaction was "No way!" I thought, *I'm too fat and too out of shape to spin. I won't be able to do it. It would be humiliating.*

Lisa persisted: "We'll go together and get coffee afterward." I never see Lisa because we are both working moms, so the chance to spend quality time with her, even if it meant facing my fears first, was worth the risk. I took a bike in the back of the room, where I couldn't be seen, and I watched Lisa killing it in the front row. I couldn't finish the class, but I felt pretty great about just showing up. We had coffee afterward.

It was pure joy to be with my friend. I realized on the way home that I felt happy. We made it our thing, to have an adult play date to spin, with coffee after.

If it hadn't been for my fitness buddy, I wouldn't have had the nerve to try spinning. I'd still be crawling up the stairs to my office with all that weight on my body and soul. Eventually, I gained the fitness and confidence to have fun spinning on my own. I made connections with the instructors and they became my surrogate fitness buddies when Lisa wasn't available. Physically, it was hard, but it was fun and I got stronger every week. It was rewarding to challenge my body a little more each time. One step at a time, one class at a time, the fat slowly came off. The "cycle" of success culminated not just in my weight loss, but when my favorite instructor, Lori, a source of inspiration and support, asked me to ride the instructor bike at her side. I'd moved all the way up from the back of the room to leading it.

The Building Blocks of Fitness

There are five building blocks to fitness—balance, strength, cardiac capacity, flexibility, and endurance. Each one needs to be equally developed. Fitness imbalance is one of the key causes of pain and injury. Organize your fitness regimen to develop each building block equally.

If you hit the treadmill for three miles at the same pace and the same incline three times a week, you are not improving cardiac capacity, endurance, balance, flexibility, or strength. You are probably maintaining a certain level of fitness, but the unfit parts of you are staying unfit. This routine isn't building anything.

So, on the Well Path, as the weeks progress, you'll slowly integrate fitness that hits on all five building blocks. Not all at once, I promise! You won't go from nothing to running a marathon! It's a gradual path, with a low incline. When some of my patients begin, they can't climb a flight of stairs. By the end of eight weeks, they're charging up mountains. Progressing slowly prevents injury and "weekend warrior syndrome." You know what that is: You're sedentary all week, and then, on the weekends, you push too hard, feel awful, get sore or hurt, and then quit fitness altogether until the next burst of motivation that won't last. My strategy for a varied, progressive routine incorporates fitness into your life bit by bit, so you won't ever feel overwhelmed.

The building blocks:

Strength. Muscles are metabolic powerhouses, so the more muscle mass you have, the better. Every muscle in your body is there for a reason. You need them to move, whether you are walking or blinking an eye. Building strong muscles also protects your bones. Every time you put strain on your muscles, your bones get stronger, too. Hence, strength training is crucial to prevent osteoporosis. Strengthening spine-supporting core muscles keeps your pouch in place and prevents back pain, a debilitating problem for a significant portion of the population.

Balance. Stumbling and falling because your balance is weak can take you out of your fitness fun. People who include balance in their fitness repertoire can right themselves before they hit the ground after stumbling. Broken bone averted.

Flexibility. Flexibility keeps your muscles, tendons, and joints supple, and actually makes you stronger because when you can stretch your muscles, they have greater capacity to contract. See how beautifully we are built? Increasing your flexibility will help you transition from rest to activity readily and with less pain. You will move quicker and recover faster.

Cardiac capacity. Your heart is a muscle, just like your bicep. If you don't exercise it, it will get weak. No one wants a weak heart. You want your heart to be able to support any activity you ask your body to do, whether it's walking up the stairs, running a 5K, or touring Paris on vacation. Cardiac fitness is the capacity of your heart to pump blood efficiently to your organs, delivering the maximum amount of oxygen and nutrients possible. If your treadmill activity keeps your heart rate at a steady eighty, you aren't increasing your cardiac fitness. A more effective method is to increase your heart rate in bursts with recovery rest periods in between, aka interval training. You don't have to run yourself into the ground! Any pace is the right pace as long as you keep moving forward.

Endurance. Who wants their body to peter out half a mile from the summit of the mountain? Not me! This is one of the most rewarding building blocks to work on because you will notice a real difference in your ability to do an activity longer or harder than you could previously. Running on a treadmill for thirty minutes at the same pace three times a week does nothing for endurance. When I work with patients on endurance, they are constantly surprised at how quickly it develops if they just push themselves a little bit longer one day a week. Being able to endure reminds them that they can be strong and vital well into their golden years.

Buddy Up

You've heard this advice before. If you're accountable to a workout buddy, you're more likely to stick with a routine. A friend will encourage you and congratulate you on your efforts. I'm a big believer in positive reinforcement. A kind word goes a long way. A stolen giggle in a serious class ups the fun factor and makes you feel like a team. There is even such a thing as healthy competition, when your workout buddy motivates you to push a little harder. Some women are intimidated to walk into a new class or to try something new on their own. But with a pal at your side? You become fearless together.

The greatest benefit to workouts with a buddy: more fun. Researchers at the University of Southern California's Department of Preventive Medicine asked their subjects, ages twenty-seven to seventy-three, to rate their happiness eight times a day, and to describe what they were doing, where, and with whom each time. The subjects who exercised at least once a week were happier than non-exercisers. And the happiest exercise sessions were those that took place outdoors with friends, partners, or coworkers. So grab a friend, get out there, and go for it.

Forget Trends

Fitness trends come and go, but your genes stay the same. A new field of research by Newtopia Laboratories has discovered that some of us lose weight only when we do high-intensity exercise (running, swimming, etc.) and some are slow-burners, releasing fat during long, slow exercise (walking, yoga, etc.). My body responds to hot yoga and endurance hiking and biking. They also happen to be the forms of exercise I enjoy the most. You will never find me in a CrossFit class, but I know plenty of people who love it, probably because it's the type of exercise their genetics respond to. We didn't all evolve from ancestors with the same type of physical prowess. It makes sense that our bodies would feel more at home with different exercises.

One-size-fits-all diet and fitness plans will always fail some of the people some of the time. I can't tell you what fitness choices are fun and efficient for you. But you can, and you will. It's the only way to integrate a sustainable fitness routine. Exercise, more so than any other C.H.A.N.G.E. category, is a very personal decision based on your age, fitness level, location, lifestyle, and preferences. Not everyone can go surfing or skiing on the weekend. Do what makes sense for your lifestyle and is fun for you, not someone else, not what you heard will "work." And don't be afraid to try something totally new, because you just might miss out on something you'll grow to be passionate about.

Go Outside and Play!

Working and living in artificial environments—with artificial air, artificial light, and artificial sounds—contributes to our hormonal imbalance. I have seen amazing emotional and physical transformations in patients I've taken hiking in the mountains outside New York City. Even the city slickers in the group clamor for a slot on these Saturday walks in the woods. Why do they love it? At our core, humans are natural beings. When we're immersed in nature, it taps into our deepest evolutionary instincts. The beauty of nature can be found anywhere, and it is *free*.

I know my advice sounds so Mommy-ish. Eat soup! Call a friend! Go play outside! But the research backs it all up. The Japanese make a special practice of *shinrin-yoku*, or forest bathing. Just walking or hiking in a forest exposes you to phytoncides, chemicals emitted by trees that improve your immune function. A fifteen-minute walk in the woods can reduce blood pressure and drop cortisol levels by 16 percent. A 2007 study of Japanese men found that a two-hour walk outside can increase the activity of cancer-fighting white blood cells by 40 percent.

Combining exercise with the great outdoors is how all of your fit friends have fun. They get it. When you're outside moving around, sucking in that fresh air and soaking up the vitamin D–producing rays of the sun, you get positive reinforcement to keep you active for longer periods of time. Think of little kids who complain about having to leave the park.

I discovered hiking or walking in the woods after I had my third child as a way to be active on the weekends with all my kids. Before then, I'd only hiked a couple times in my life. I was desperate to find something that got me out of the house, so I bought a book about hikes near New York City, harnessed my newborn to my chest, and started ticking the hikes off one weekend at a time. I discovered how easy it is to work on your fitness for hours at a stretch when you are in nature. Climbing over rocks and jumping over streams works all the building blocks of fitness and, most important, it rejuvenated my spirit. Instant antidepressant. Compare that to hitting the gym, where the whole idea is to get in, do your thing, and get out as quickly as possible.

Building Block Checkpoints

There's a lot of fitness advice out there to wade through. I have spent years following fitness trends and research. I've consulted with some of the best fitness experts around. If you tried to absorb all the information available, it'd be a full-time job. So, unless fitness is your job, don't bother trying. Just remember the five building blocks. Pay attention to working on them. To make sure you are, ask yourself the following questions. If the answers are "yes," you're on the right path.

> Did I go a little farther this week in my fitness activity?
> Can I lift a heavier weight or hold a yoga position longer this week?
> Are my muscles a little sore after strength training?
> If I stand on one foot or walk a straight line, is my balance better?
> Can I deepen my stretches?
> When my heart is pumping, can I breath better?
> Does my heart rate recover more quickly between intervals?

If the answer is "no" to any of them, you need to push yourself a little bit harder until you see a change. You will experience some uncomfortable feelings both physically and emotionally, but I encourage you to acknowledge the discomfort and allow progress to happen. Discomfort does not mean acute pain, light-headedness, shortness of breath, or chest tightness. It means work, sweat, and muscle fatigue. Progress by inches, not yards, and eventually you'll say "yes" to these challenges every week.

Take It Easy

A lot of women think that you have to exert yourself like a maniac to burn fat. Not true. Working out at a medium intensity for a longer stretch of time can be just as beneficial or more beneficial than exercising strenuously for a shorter period. A study published in a 2012 article in *Physiological Reviews* showed that longer-duration fixed-intensity exercise boosted lipolytic rate, a measure for how effectively you metabolize fat for energy. If you want to access long-term storage fat—the stuff on your belly and butt—try to include one exercise session per week that lasts two hours or more at a steady pace, like a long vigorous walk with friends on the beach or a bike ride on a long path.

If you tend to go hard and flame out, it's a destructive pattern. Yo-yo exercising has the same impact on the body as yo-yo dieting. Over time, you wind up gaining fat each up-and-down cycle. Going back and forth between bouts of intense over-the-top exercise, to less exercise or none, signals your body to hold on to the fat for when you'll go hard again (if ever).

Last January, I put this theory to the test. I took twenty-five women through my program, and (insanely?) volunteered to each one to be their fitness buddy. Yes, that meant I would be exercising about fifteen times a week for eight weeks. At first, I started off pretty strong. I was sore for a while but that faded. I got in the swing of doing new classes, and things I hadn't done in a while.

After a week or two, my body started insisting I conserve energy. I found myself phoning it in at each class. The only joy I got out of it was being with my buddies. I had no time to rest. I ate well but didn't change my diet much or increase my calories. During eight weeks of exercising two or three hours per day, I didn't lose any fat. When I finally dropped my fitness frequency to normal—three yoga classes a week—I promptly gained five pounds. I also injured my shoulder, and I never get injured.

Overexercise threw me out of homeostasis. In order to preserve energy for that insane level of activity, my body held on to the fat by slowing my normal processes down. Contrast that intensity with going on a weekly walk in the woods. My body becomes a fat-burning machine, even though I'm "exercising" all day. The pace is slow and steady. I push myself just enough to keep up with the challenge. I stretch morning and night. There are some bouts of intensity, but then

I rest. For nonathletes, unsustainable overexercising does not work long-term for fat loss or fitness capacity. In fact, it can cause both injury and weight gain when you crash and quit, which is inevitable.

Of course, intensity is subjective. Your low-intensity might be someone else's limit. Whatever high or low intensity means to you, don't push yourself beyond your limits. If you're after fat loss, slow and steady wins the race. Remember, whatever exercise is fun and doable for you long-term is going to be your ticket. Keep in mind the five building blocks plus joy, and you'll have a winning combination.

Doing the Best You Can Do in the Context of Your Life Is Good Enough

Emily, thirty-two, was newly engaged and came to me to get in great shape before her wedding and in anticipation of one day getting pregnant. In the past, she'd tried many diets and trendy exercise routines but couldn't stick with anything. She worked at a high-pressure job and found that her work and social life got in the way of her fitness and healthy eating.

She told me she had three or four drinks whenever she went out.

"How often do you go out?" I asked.

"Four nights a week? Five?"

Emily was having between twelve and twenty drinks a week. No wonder she couldn't seem to lose any weight. Her liver was otherwise occupied filtering all that alcohol and couldn't efficiently process fat.

She started the Well Path, cut back on the drinking, and made the soups. She went rock climbing with me twice a week. For a while. Then life took over. Her job got intense and she was working an extra twenty hours a week. Nutrifying her meals went out the window and she missed a few workouts. "It was a hectic time with a lot of balls in the air. I lost track of the Path going out to lunches and working so hard with clients and meetings," she said. "But then I would go home and have a soup for dinner. I'd remember to have lemon water in the morning. Just keeping up with a few of the small steps got me back on track. I realized that I had to be forgiving and realistic. Some weeks, I'd be super-psyched to do it all. Other weeks, I couldn't do anything. But it was all okay.

"I worked out some fundamentals about what being healthy means," she said. "Compared to some of the other women I met doing the Well Path, I hadn't taken my nutrition or fitness to a higher level. But I was allowed to feel good about the changes I did make that I know I'll do forever."

I congratulated Emily on her self-awareness and realistic attitude about wellness. You're not in a competition or a race. You're hiking your hike, ever mindful of what you can do, and doing it to the best of your ability. She nodded and said, "I with I'd had this revelation sooner. Why didn't I change my mind-set earlier?"

Ha! I wish I'd had this revelation at thirty-two!

Becoming mindful and forgiving is a breakthrough. Congratulations to Emily and to every woman who learns this valuable insight at any age.

Kick It Up a Notch Once in a While

To lose inches, you have to liberate the contents of the fat cell *and* sweep the fatty acids away into the circulation to be used by the body. You already know how you must have robust blood vessels in adipose tissue—connective tissue comprised of fat cells—to mobilize fat. Moderate-intensity exercise is a powerful stimulator of blood flow through your adipose tissue. Adipose tissue blood flow can double during moderate exercise if you are *not* obese. If you are obese, it's harder to access those fat storage areas with exercise, which is why I've asked you to do all of those other circulation builders, such as skin brushing. High-intensity exercise has been proven to sustain fat liberation in the post-exercise afterburn period.

So, on the Well Path, you will be mixing up the slow and steady with some high-intensity exercise. Don't worry if you don't understand what this is. I will guide you. It will not be too hard. It will be just hard enough to keep you moving forward in a fun, sustainable, and successful way.

I want you to shift your concept of exercise. Exercise isn't just about weight loss: it's about building strength, endurance, flexibility, and having fun. It's about reducing stress and gaining energy. Weight loss *will* happen if you go outside and play for the right reasons. Changing the way you look at exercise is the most powerful thing you can do to break the cycle of fitness failure and get out of the yo-yo exercise rut.

Free Your Fat

I get asked all the time about combining nutrition and exercise for maximum fat loss. It's an interesting question, and there is a formula that I'm going to share with you below. But even more important than planning how to eat in combination with fitness is exercising to compensate for bingeing. The "I'll eat this pie tonight and work out twice as hard tomorrow" phenomenon is a losing strategy, but not in the way you want. After a big meal, you have what's called a postprandial dip, the insulin response that makes you tired. My kids call it the JAMS, or "just ate, must sleep." Exercising after such a meal trains the body not to metabolize stored fat, but to go for the glycogen stored in muscles instead. How often do you actually get up early and do the compensation workout anyway? Honestly? Besides which, inconsistent exercise will trigger your survival mode metabolism and counterintuitively *increase* fat storage.

It's a wiser strategy to exercise *before* the splurge. Storage of fat after exercise is decreased due to afterburn, the body's revved-up metabolism that is particularly speedy for ten to twelve hours post-workout. I understand that you can't always plan when you're going to overeat. But just having the knowledge that the old way of responding to extra-calorie intake with exercise will backfire might turn the switch in your head to not splurge unless you've already exercised that day.

Now, to the question of how to combine eating with exercise to guarantee that you will power your workout with fat for energy: You want this to happen, obviously, to shrink fat cells. It'll also supercharge your workout. Fatty acid energy yields 133 percent more punch than glucose. Not only will you lose inches, you'll bounce off the walls.

The Free Fat Formula helps you to operate with greater efficiency.

Up to one hour before a workout: Eat a meal or snack of complex carbs, lean protein, fiber, and healthy fat, such as steel-cut oatmeal with almond milk; half a banana, pecans, and chia seeds; or sprouted grain bread, organic cheese, an egg, and half a tomato. Why carbs pre-workout? When insulin is slightly elevated, cortisol goes down. That's a good thing: Cortisol breaks down muscle tissue for energy. Lowering cortisol with carbs primes your body to liberate fat for energy by the time you start your workout (and will continue to do so during your workout and afterward).

The 75/25 Workout: Work out split between moderate intensity (75 percent) and interval cardio and/or power building (25 percent). Interval training is short bursts of high-intensity cardio (running as fast as you can for sixty seconds) or power building (doing ten pushups), followed by short periods of rest (after a one-minute sprint, walk for thirty seconds; after ten pushups, lie flat with your face on the carpet, gasping for breath, which is what I do). A half hour of high-intensity interval training will liberate and mobilize twice as much fat as an hour of sustained medium-intensity exercise, but bookending with moderate exercise increases the circulation in adipose tissue to mobilize released fat. Interestingly, many fitness classes are set up like this. Warm up with moderate intensity, increase to high-intensity intervals at the end, then go back to moderate and cool down. Let's say that you are taking up running; for the first twenty minutes, run at a moderately intense pace where you can talk and control your breathing and your heart isn't bursting out of your chest. Sprint for a minute, then slow down and jog until you recover; repeat the pattern until you're done. Then jog to cool down. If you are incorporating strength training into this, alternate sprints for jumping squats or pushups or running up stairs. You get the idea.

Immediately after workout: A liquid form of protein and carbs, like a protein shake or a green juice that includes plant proteins like kale and chia seeds. In liquid form, it's easily digestible. You need the protein for rebuilding muscles after the workout. The carbs remind the body that resources are plentiful, and it doesn't have to hold on to fat.

Two hours post-workout: A main meal of protein, healthy fat, and carbs, *plus* sixteen ounces of water. Eating a couple of hours post-workout is like throwing fuel on a fire. It sends the message to the adipocytes that they can keep leaking fat for energy. A huge glass of water will help move it along.

Bedtime: To fall asleep, I mentioned a bedtime snack of protein plus carbs. At the end of a workout day, your body craves more nutrients to do its nighttime repair and rebuilding and generate the right hormones to do it all over again the day after tomorrow. Your bedtime snack on workout days should be a healthy fat with slow-digesting protein (nuts, nut butter, avocado, hummus).

PART THREE

The Well Path in Action

12

Prep Week

When women say "The diet starts tomorrow," it's already over. Changes that are too abrupt and too dramatic will not take root. You can't rush into the rest of your life. But if you make C.H.A.N.G.E. gradually, you'll slowly adapt a healthy lifestyle that is sustainable.

Lifelong changes happen on the Well Path, and they will unfurl at a steady pace. As the old saying goes, it takes a month to make or break a habit. It also takes a month to regenerate a cell, balance hormones, and lengthen your telomeres. Every step on the Well Path has been calibrated over years of practice with patients so that they are achievable, flexible, and sustainable. After being on the Path for eight weeks, patients say they are on a new path for life.

But first, before you can implement the C.H.A.N.G.E. to come, you have to prepare yourself mentally, emotionally, and practically. Just as you wouldn't leave for a trip without packing and mapping out the itinerary beforehand, you need to prepare for the Path, too.

Prep Week is a time for you to shop, think, learn, and mentally prepare before you begin the process of easing your body back into homeostasis. By cozying up to the strategies and getting excited about the small-yet-seismic changes you're about to enact, you'll be priming yourself for success.

Many of my patients have noticed that simply preparing for the Well Path shifted their attitude about nutrition and fitness.

Understanding why past efforts had failed, and how they can affect real, lasting change helped their bodies relax. That sense of relief affected their hormonal feedback loop for the better, allowing homeostasis to begin. Changing your mind-set is essential. I'm going to ask you to be patient before beginning your journey . . . for a few more days, and a few more pages, to ensure that you are prepared for success.

Awareness

The theme of Prep Week is awareness. You will shine a new light on your hunger patterns and activity frequency. Connecting to your body will help to rekindle a lost awareness of your health. Tuning in is critical to your success, so don't let fear of what you might discover block you from these exercises. There is no judgment, no shame, just awareness. Awareness is what gives you the power to change the trajectory of your health. If finding balance is the goal, the first step must be becoming mindful of your imbalances. Tracking your inactivity and keeping a Hunger Diary will trigger those "aha" moments.

During Prep Week, you will:

Collect a few Well Path tools

Start keeping hunger and inactivity logs

Enlist a workout buddy or two

Plan your exercise schedule for the next week

Think about how to nutrify your favorite meals

Make two soups

That's it.

Well Path Don'ts

The following are useless habits from a previous life. You don't need them anymore.

Don't stress. During the entire prep period, you must wrap your mind around the fact that you are NOT about to embark on a diet that will make you eliminate food groups or leave you hungry. As I've said many times, dieting makes you fat, and even thinking about preparing to diet releases stress hormones that throw your body off balance.

Don't smoke. You already know smoking is bad for you, but it also ages your skin and throws your body out of homeostasis, hampering weight loss. If you are a smoker, this is the time to cut back or quit cold turkey.

Don't use artificial sweeteners. Your body registers anything sweet as a call to release insulin, resulting in the same fat-hoarding hormonal environment as if you were eating real sugar. If you must sweeten something, I would prefer you eat organic raw sugar, agave, or honey, which at least have no added chemicals.

Don't skip ahead. Each step builds on the preceding step to ensure seamless integration into your life and ultimate sustainability. If you aren't able to start a particular step right away, don't worry. Just start it as soon as you can and then follow the natural progression of the steps. I have had patients start one strategy from Week One in Week Four. I tell them: Just keep moving forward. This isn't just for eight weeks; it's for life.

What You Need to Get Started

When I work with patients in my practice, I give them a starter kit for Prep Week that includes:

A dry brush. At any pharmacy or online, you can find a natural-bristle dry body brush for less than $20. It is a tiny expense for life-changing benefits. If a plastic surgeon said to you, "For twenty bucks, I'll make your legs/arms/belly look better," I think you would happily hand over the money. Well, for that same $20, you can buy a high-quality dry brush and make your body better yourself.

A fitness tracker. A fitness tracker is a useful tool, but completely optional. You can also download a free pedometer app to your phone. The iPhone 5 and 6 come pre-loaded with the Health app, which tracks your steps during both inactive and active times. Or, like me, you can just use a good old-fashioned watch to time your activity and inactivity. If you are inclined to buy a fitness tracker, I like the Jawbone brand, because it is simple to use. The most basic versions have a pedometer and sleep monitor, which is what you'd use on the Path Program through my practice.

A small thermos. Just enough to hold 2 cups of soup. If you have one lying around the house somewhere, dig it out. You'll use it to make your soup lunches portable.

A small folder. The folder is dedicated to your hunger and inactivity logs. You can download and print a sample Hunger Diary page for each week from my website at www.thewellpathbook.com. The act of writing by hand helps you connect your thoughts and behavior with your physical experience (aka biofeedback), which is the key to integrating mindfulness.

A pound of lemons. These will be used to make your morning hot lemon water.

A soup pot. I recommend an 8-quart capacity, preferably with as wide/thick a base as possible to evenly cook the large quantities of veggies. I prefer a nonstick bottom for ease of cooking and cleanup.

Track Your Inactivity

The goal in Prep Week is to evaluate where you are *now*. If you opted to use technology to track your fitness, learn how to use your app, your fitness tracker, or your watch. Start your Daily Inactivity

Worksheets, record the minutes of inactive time (sitting on your butt or lying down; don't count sleep) and active time (when you are moving and on your feet). For example, if you get in your car and drive thirty minutes to work, include the time you started the inactivity and the time you stopped the inactivity. See the sample worksheet below.

Type of Inactivity	Time of Start and End of Inactivity	Total Inactive Time
Sitting at breakfast	8 a.m.–8:15 a.m.	15 min
Driving car to work	8:30 a.m.–9:30 a.m.	60 min
Sitting at desk	9:45 a.m.–11 a.m.	75 min
Sitting at meeting	11:10 a.m.–2 p.m.	170 min
Sitting at desk	2:05 p.m.–5 p.m.	175 min
Driving home	5:10 p.m.–6:10 p.m.	60 min
Dinner in bed/ watching TV	7 p.m.–9 p.m.	120 min

Total Time: 11.25 hrs

At the end of each day, tally the daily total from the Inactivity Worksheet (download from our website at www.thewellpathbook.com) and transfer to the chart below.

If you are tracking your steps, record how many you take in a fifteen-minute active period of time during the course of your day. For example, if you don't sit down the first fifteen minutes after arriving home from work, record how many steps that is.

Fifteen-minute step count: _____

Inactivity Chart

Prep Week	Total Inactive Time	Total Active Time
Monday _____		_____
Tuesday _____		_____
Wednesday _____		_____
Thursday _____		_____
Friday _____		_____
Saturday _____		_____
Sunday _____		_____

Track Your Hunger

It's important not to react to your hunger patterns just yet. Begin to notice your hunger so that you can record it accurately. If you start to notice some interesting patterns, great. Your goal is awareness. Notice, but don't judge. Observe, but don't obsess. Fill out one diary per day for the week. For example:

Time of Day	Hunger Rating 1–5
7:45 a.m.	3
8:30 a.m.	5
10 a.m.	5
12 p.m.	4
3 p.m.	5 plus
7 p.m.	4
9 p.m.	4

Experiment with Your Favorite Breakfast

Most of the women I treat have been so fixated on following some plan's version of breakfast for years that they have a hard time answering when I ask them what they like to eat for breakfast. On the Well Path we're interested in what food you genuinely love, and figuring out how to nutrify that. So this week I want you to think about your favorite breakfast, and experiment with ways to add the Four F's— fruit, fat, fiber, and fuel—to it. For example, if your favorite breakfast of all time is . . .

Pancakes with Butter and Syrup

If you eat a stack of pancakes without nutrifying them, your body will be starving by 10 a.m. But if you add the Four F's to them, you'll feel satisfied with half the amount you usually eat.

Add fresh or frozen fruit to the mix, or in place of syrup. I like to soften blueberries in a pan with a little water and a tablespoon of syrup. The fruit is sweet enough, and the taste of the maple is still there.

Add healthy fat by putting ground walnuts or pecans in the mix and by cooking with less coconut oil instead of more butter.

Add fiber by swapping the boxed mix you grew up using and substituting a Bob's Red Mill Organic High Fiber Pancake Mix (buy on Amazon or in a grocery store). Throw a teaspoon of flax seeds or chia seeds into the mix for extra fiber (and fuel). Grind up some buckwheat and substitute 50/50 with the pancake mix.

Add fuel by adding cooked quinoa or an extra egg to the batter. (See more suggestions on our website.)

Choose what you LIKE, nutrify it, and you will eat less volume because the food will be filling and satisfying.

Yogurt Cup

When women tell me they eat a "healthy" fat-free yogurt with the fruit on the bottom, I cringe. Those packaged yogurt cups have virtually no nutrients and a ton of added sugar or artificial sweeteners. If you love yogurt, make these changes and you will never go back to that fat-free nonsense:

Start with a plain Greek yogurt, which has more protein and less sugar than regular yogurt. Low-fat and organic is the best combination.

Add fruit, fresh or frozen, not that goop at the bottom that's basically sugar and artificial flavor.

Add fat by using plain Greek low-fat yogurt, not the "flavored" fat-free kind. Eat fat to lose fat. Fat free is bad for your body and brain. Nuts and seeds can also be added for healthy fat. I've even added a quarter of an avocado, hemp seeds, black beans, and a little Sriracha for a savory version.

Add fiber and fuel by sprinkling in some chia seeds, nuts, or grains. I keep some cooked quinoa in the refrigerator and throw ¼ cup into my yogurt.

Hard-Boiled Egg Whites and a Piece of Dry Whole-Wheat Toast

The saddest breakfast on Earth.

Add fruit. Antioxidant-rich fruit like oranges or berries will put some color on your plate.

Add fat by eating the yolk. By not eating the yolk, you're only saving about fifty calories. It's not going to make much of a difference, and the fat and protein in the yolk will fill you up. The yolk is full of nutrients. Adding a quarter of an avocado to your toast is another way to add healthy fat.

Add fiber by substituting the factory-packaged whole-wheat toast with gluten-free ancient grain or brown rice toast. Ezekiel brand sprouted grain or spelt or brown rice bread is available at any Whole Foods, Trader Joe's, and many supermarket chains, or you can order through an online grocery store.

Add fuel by eating the yolk. Hemp or flax seeds taste delicious on eggs. If you like cheese, you can experiment with a combo of nutritional yeast and cayenne. One of my favorite combos is 2 eggs, black beans, hemp seeds, and Sriracha.

Instant Oatmeal from a Packet with Skim Milk

I bet you can already guess what I'm going to say about this. But, just to be clear:

Add fruit by throwing in fresh or frozen berries. (My freezer is packed with a variety so I don't get caught without fruit.) Don't use raisins unless you make them yourself, and then use them sparingly because the sugar is very concentrated. Sometimes I chop up homemade raisins very small so that I get a taste in every bite, but use a lot less.

Add fat, and if you prefer cow's milk, make your oatmeal with 1- or 2-percent milk and get rid of the skim. Almond milk, hemp milk, and coconut milk are also good options. This is a great place to easily start substituting nonanimal calories into your routine.

Add fiber by using steel-cut oatmeal. Using half quinoa or buckwheat groats with half oatmeal raises your fiber quotient.

Add fuel with nuts and seeds. I love pumpkin seeds in my oatmeal. Any seed or nut goes well with oatmeal. Again, if you chop the add-ins fine, you will use less with just as much flavor.

These are just a few examples of the many ways you can add the Four F's to your breakfasts this week. Make a field trip to your favorite supermarket to explore what's available, or check out a new supermarket that offers healthier options. Go online and check out your go-to add-ins, like flax seeds and chia seeds. They can easily be delivered to you if you can't find them locally. There are more recipe ideas and links on our website.

Decide on Three Fun Exercise Options

What exercise is fun for you? Have you recently taken a class or seen someone doing something athletic that made you think, *I should try that?* Explore the options that make sense for your location and lifestyle. Whatever it is, it must be convenient and sustainable. Driving two towns away at 5 a.m. to catch a spinning class may not be sustainable. Go online and do a search of gyms, community centers, YMCAs, fitness studios, and recreational sports leagues in your area. Jot down your ideas below and start researching when and where you can find your fun!

Fitness Idea #1: _____

Fitness Idea #2: _____

Fitness Idea #3: _____

Find Your Workout Buddy

If you're committed to working out with someone, you're a lot less likely to bail at the last minute or find an excuse to not show up. I've noticed that women are often all too willing to shortchange themselves, but they wouldn't dream of shortchanging someone else. A buddy prevents you from letting yourself down. Eventually, if your partner can't keep a workout date, you'll be confident enough to go alone. You'll say, "I'm not going to let myself down. *I'm* the priority."

Working out with others also ratchets up the fun factor. When I did a belly dancing class with a friend I was horrible, but I've never laughed so hard in my life and I got a great workout. Having a partner removes the stress, self-consciousness, and anxiety about walking into a new class. You'll relax and get more out of the fitness itself, and feel wonderful while celebrating your hard work afterward.

So who will it be? Who wants to get on the Well Path with you? In the best of all worlds, you'll line up a few buddies so you have backups. Don't be shy about asking, as supporting each other is one of the most loved parts of this program by my patients. People are only too willing to participate, and are thrilled to be asked to join.

Workout Buddy: _____

Backup Buddy: _____

Backup Buddy: _____

Make Soup!

Take a few moments to turn to page 249 and peruse the soup recipes. Decide which two soups you'll make before you start the Path. If you are doing the Path with a buddy, get together and make two soups each for double the variety the first week. Each recipe makes twelve 2-cup servings. Portion out the individual servings in freezer/microwave-safe containers, and freeze all but one week's worth, which will go into the fridge. Lunch is now easy, fresh, and nutrified.

Soup Choice #1:_____

Soup Choice #2:_____

Some people just don't enjoy cooking and feel nervous about this step. Here are a few quick tips that I have found helpful for making good soup:

1. Measure. You must have proper measuring instruments: a set of measuring spoons and dry and wet measuring cups.

2. Chop/mince/dice: Go online to our website and look at a basic knifework tutorial. Become familiar with the difference so that your veggies cook properly.

3. Check out your spice rack. If you're going to substitute fresh herbs for dried, make sure you have what you need in advance. Look up the equivalent measures for fresh versus dried so you don't accidentally add too much when you're in the throes of cooking.

Why Soup Is SOUPER!!!

Soup is universally appealing. I've never met anyone who didn't like
soup.

Soup forces you to eat slowly.

Soup is hydrating.

Soup has endless variety.

Soup can be made ahead in enormous quantities and stored.

Soup keeps all the nutrients and goodies in the broth that would be
lost if you cooked veggies and then transferred them to the plate.

Soup is easily digestible.

Soup is warm, and warmed food has more flavor.

Soup is a go-to lunch, eliminating decision-making, supplying you
with the most nutritious meal of the day to fuel your afternoon,
and keeping you from feeling deprived at dinnertime.

Soup is transportable. Have thermos, will travel. It can be eaten
anywhere.

Soup is affordable. You'll definitely save money by not buying lunch
every day.

Soup does not have the stigma of a "diet" food. Your family and
colleagues will want to steal your soup, so you can be proud that
you made something that everyone thinks is delicious. You have
been warned!

Prep Week Questionnaire

You've spent the week getting ready, mentally and logistically, to get
on the Well Path. The very last part of Prep Week is answering the
following question:

What is my body fat percentage? _____

OR, if you can't get your body fat tested (your primary care physician or gym should be able to do it), choose the one pair of jeans in your closet that you are closest to fitting into. If you want to take a photo of yourself, that's great. Sometimes you only know how far you have come by looking back at where you came from.

Rate the following from 1 to 5 (1 being the lowest and 5 being the highest):

Energy:_____

Sex drive:_____

Sleep quality: _____

Aches and pains: _____

Bowel movements: _____

Fitness:_____

Mood: _____

Stress coping: _____

Concentration: _____

Memory: _____

Move Your Health to the Top of Your Priorities List

My patient Denise is a forty-seven-year-old working mother who takes care of everything but herself. She is one of the loveliest, smartest, and most hardworking women I have ever met, but her brightness was dulling because she'd been sidelining her well-being for years, going from managing one crisis to the next. Her life just kept blowing up, and Denise rushed in to triage constantly. When she came to me, she was stressed out and looking for a way back to being active and feeling healthy again. "I used to be this super-fit, super-healthy girl," she said. "I totally lost my way. I want to reconnect to the person I used to be. And not eat so much! My portion size is out of control."

It was hard for her to get away to take a class or make soup. But she persisted, and her husband stepped up to help. She resurrected a gym in her basement and her husband freed her up from responsibilities so she could use it regularly. Now, after two months on the Path, she reports real improvement. Even her cravings for comfort food have abated. "Now, when I look at a cream-filled pastry, all I can think is that the sugar will attack my mouth. I'll feel bad, physically, if I eat that. I crave my lemon water. I jump up to walk the dog instead of telling the kids to do it. I travel for my new job, and pack fruit in my suitcase. I have a pound of lemons in my carry-on!"

Along with losing seven pounds of fat and fourteen years off her metabolic age, Denise feels empowered. "No one can tell you that you can't jump right back to being your best self," she said. "I was able to do it gradually, and it wasn't hard! I know I can sustain it, too. I'm just going to keep going, doing what I've been doing. Easy."

13.

Week One

You're ready to go! You've got all your tools. You've got your soups. Now it's time to take your first steps on the Path.

The whole premise of this program is to make simple, sustainable, enjoyable changes that will gently bring your body back to homeostasis. With all of the C.H.A.N.G.E.s working seamlessly together, your body can achieve balance and health. No matter what is happening at work or at home, if you follow the Path, you will fortify yourself so that you can sail through whatever life throws at you. C.H.A.N.G.E. works *within* your life while you gain energy, strengthen your muscles, and lose fat. So tell your body that it's going to feast (instead of famine), feel strong (instead of stressed), and be nurtured (instead of be neglected), and then do the work and watch it thrive.

The theme of this week is excitement. Get psyched to let your body do what it's supposed to do instead of fighting against it. Be thrilled to have fun! You can do more, be more, feel more, and experience it all with a strong, vital, energized body and mind.

How the Well Path works: Each week, you'll incorporate one activity from each C.H.A.N.G.E. category into your life. You'll have all week to practice the strategies so you can build on them in subsequent weeks. Practice does not make perfect, it makes habit.

If I can give something to put in your backpack on this journey, let me give you the freedom to be imperfect. Doing the best you can is good enough (are you sick of hearing that yet?). When I take women through the Well Path in New York, I remind them that perfectionism is sabotage. I tell them my own stories of failure. Guess what? Everyone fails. Getting over perfectionism years ago set me free to be the best person I can be. I don't worry about my legs looking perfect. They propel me up mountains just fine. I don't worry about the big scar across the bridge of my nose. It got there when I dared to push myself, fell flat on my face, got up, and kept going. I don't worry about my patients knowing that I, like them, have a mountain in front of me. Support is a two-way street. With their support, I know I can keep climbing. Whenever you feel like you aren't measuring up, just picture me right there next to you, reminding you that all you have to do is put one foot in front of the other. On our website, we have a community of women just like you who have come together in support of one another.

C.H.A.N.G.E. Strategies for Week One

Circulation

Week One Goal:

Drink 8 ounces of warm water with lemon first thing every morning.

Heat opens up the blood flow to the intestines and the lemon pushes your body's pH balance toward alkaline, which decreases blood-flow-blocking inflammation. When blood is flowing to the intestines, gut absorption is functioning optimally, and every one of your cells is happier. You want your intestines to absorb nutrients like a greedy sponge to feed your cells all of the wonderful food you will be eating.

That's it. You should have bought a pound of lemons during Prep Week.

Step-by-Step:

If you weigh less than 150 pounds, use half a lemon; if you weigh
more, use the whole lemon.

Slice the lemon and squeeze the juice into a mug or glass (rinds are notoriously covered in nasty stuff, so don't drop them in too). Add warm water. Drink this before anything else hits that tummy—even coffee.

Hunger

Week One Goals:

- Keep up the Hunger Diary. Recording your hunger patterns increases awareness and decreases emotion. In fact, your Hunger Diary will eventually serve to increase your sensation of real hunger in its earliest stages, giving you space to be mindful of how best to respond to it. Remember, hunger is just a physiological response. It's not an alarm bell or an air raid siren. It is your body reminding you to refuel with nutrients.

- Use a visual representation for the hunger signal. Use an image of mass transportation that you can drive or fly in and out of your vision. Every time you are hungry this week, see that image moving into your space, and after you eat, visualize it moving away. Right now picture that airplane or bus completely empty. Don't skip this step even if it feels a little silly, because we will be building onto it later.

Hunger signal image:_____

Activity

Everyone has a routine, and routines are never easy to change. I know having a routine makes me feel comfortable and at ease with my day. Could I have a "better" routine? I'm sure I could, but it'd be hard to comply with, given the locked-down schedule I have to adhere to with three kids and an appointment-based business. If I tried to change my routine drastically, even with good intentions, it wouldn't work. I'd set myself up to feel like a failure—not good, and not part of the Path.

For example, I used to beat myself up for not getting up earlier in the morning to knock out my exercise. That would certainly be "better" in someone's book. Well, guess what? I can't do it. I'm not a morning exerciser. I want to sleep until the last possible moment. If I tried to get up an hour earlier just to exercise, I would fail. So I don't even try. Does that make me a failure? No, it makes me aware of what doesn't work for me.

This is where I want you to be. What good is a "better" routine if it doesn't work with your life or makes you feel bad about yourself? It's worthless. In the best of all worlds, you establish a good routine that's effortless to stick to.

Any good routine includes activity. Where can you fit in more activity? Can the activity become part of your routine, like dropping the kids off at school and arriving at work? Making this happen will require you to make it a priority, plan, and experiment until it becomes routine.

Remind yourself how many steps you take in fifteen minutes of active time if you are using a step tracker.

Fifteen-minute active step count: _____

Week One Goal:

Map your daily routine.

What time do you wake up? What time do you leave the house? How long is your commute? What time do you get to work or school? Do you take breaks during the day? When's lunch, dinner, snack time? When do you leave for home? Go to bed? You get the idea. Map it all out.

Look for opportunities in your routine to add activity. Your inactivity log, pedometer app, fitness tracker, and daily calendar can help you analyze this routine and find the space to easily add fifteen minutes of non-exercise activity. The fifteen minutes can be in one chunk or you can sneak them in piecemeal, adding to an activity you're already doing or adding something new.

For years, I walked to the office from my apartment. Then we moved and I started to drive to work. I parked less than a block away from my office and perfectly timed my arrival. I was proud of my efficiency, but I sacrificed activity for convenience. Boy, did I sacrifice. Within a month, I gained five pounds. My solution was to park at a garage two miles away from the office. Now, no matter the weather, I walk two miles back and forth through Central Park to work. Not only did I lose the weight without one drop of sweat, I arrived at work and home calmer and happier for having put in thirty minutes of activity before and after my workday. I need and deserve this activity. Sometimes we have to alter our world ever so slightly to do the hardest thing possible—make ourselves a priority. Find your routine, prioritize yourself, and stick with it. Everyone in your life will benefit.

Wherever you find your fifteen minutes, ask yourself if you can do it every day at the same time. It's about integration, forming a new habit. Fifteen added minutes of activity a day gives you thirty minutes of body benefit by reducing inactive time by fifteen minutes as well. That's a thirty-minute swing toward increasing your BMR.

When will you add fifteen minutes of activity to your everyday routine?

_____

Daily steps average for the week: _____

Nutrition

Be calm. Eat on.

As I hope I've made clear, I don't believe in eliminating what people *like* to eat. Nutrifying your meals so they satisfy your body on a cellular level is the key to feeding yourself on the Well Path. Being mindful of the Big Ideas regarding food, you will learn to choose nutrient-dense over calorie-dense. Try to eat less animal calories. Cook more. Eat whole, seasonal unprocessed food. Every week on the Path, you will prepare a soup recipe for your daily lunch.

Week One Goals:

Eat a 2-cup portion of soup every day for lunch. If that doesn't work, have it for dinner. Have a half-portion for a snack. If you can't heat it up in the middle of the day, break out your thermos and fill it with hot soup in the morning. It'll still be hot at lunchtime.

Establish a soup day. I have Souper Sunday. I have a dedicated time that I refuse to sideline, no matter what comes up. I shop for my ingredients on Saturday and then make soup on Sunday. My family knows that this is sacrosanct. If you'd rather soup on Wednesday, fine. But pick the same day to shop and soup each week. This should become routine and nonnegotiable.

Prepare snacks for the week. During Prep Week, you thought about ways to nutrify your favorite breakfasts and have been trying out your ideas. This week, shift the focus to snacks. I recommend making snack bags of one-hundred-calorie portions for the whole week (I like to do this while my soup is simmering). That way you'll be mindful about snacking, and you'll have great options when you need them and be less likely to eat unhealthy options or go hungry. Make as many as needed so you're always prepared.

A Word about Treats

Chocolate is *not* a snack. A cookie is not a snack. Chocolate is a treat. Cookies are a treat. Treats are great. I love treats. I used to love it when my father asked, "Who wants to go get a treat?" on random nights after dinner. We would get in the car and go find a treat. It was special because it wasn't every day. Don't deny yourself a treat here and there, but don't eat it when you're hungry. Snacks are the fuel bridge between your bigger meals. Be mindful of their value to your body. Enjoy treats in moderation to prevent the growth of neural pathways that lead to food addiction. If you treat it like a treat, by the end of the program, you will be surprised how long a bar of chocolate, a tub of ice cream, or a tin of cookies sticks around your kitchen.

Some snack suggestions:

Nuts. Nuts offer fat and fiber. Throw in some seeds and a little dried fruit (not too much!), and you've got the Four F's in one bag. Measure it the first time so you know for sure how much you are putting into your snack bag.

Popcorn. It's packed with fiber and will fill your stomach nicely. Buy non-GMO organic popcorn. Corn is one of the most pesticide-laden and modified foods we eat in this country. I like Bob's Red Mill brand. Pop it yourself: Turn on the stove to medium heat. Put a pot on the burner and drop in 1 teaspoon of organic coconut oil. Wait for it to liquefy. Put ½ cup of kernels into the pot. Cover tightly. Wait for the first few kernels to pop, and then gently shake the pot over the heat until the popping stops.

Fruit. A portable piece of fruit like an apple or banana is the easiest snack to prepare. Nature has already packaged it for you. Ideally, you'll combine fruit with a little fat and protein, like a small piece of cheese, raw almond butter, or a handful of cashews. But it is also just fine to have on its own.

Soup! I always prepare a few 1-cup soup portions to have as snacks, too. Great for after dinner. A hot, comforting bit of love before bed.

Which day will you make soup? _____

Soup recipe #3: _____

Snack #1: _____

Snack #2: _____

Snack #3: _____

General Health

This week, it's all about sleep.

Sleep is step one toward balance and homeostasis. When people say, "I'll sleep when I'm dead," I always think, *Yeah, it'll be sooner than later.* You can't turn back the clock on aging without adequate rest. Your cells and mood will suffer. Your metabolism will crawl and your telomeres will shrink.

Week One Goals:

Turn off all screens one hour before sleep.

Choose a reasonable bedtime.

Set a weeknight bedtime that's only fifteen minutes earlier than your current one. Weekends can vary slightly, but it is best to be as consistent as possible. Getting overly ambitious and saying, "I'll be in bed by nine every night" might trigger anxiety-related insomnia when you don't fall asleep right away. Gently ease into an earlier evening ritual.

Stocking up on some sleep tools, like an old-fashioned alarm clock to replace your phone, a sleep mask, and ear plugs can go a long way toward successful rest. Some people also find it helpful to take a melatonin thirty minutes before bedtime, or sprinkle lavender oil on their pillow.

Reasonable bedtime: _____

Exercise

Exercise should be fun. Its purpose is to build your strength, endurance, cardiac capacity, flexibility, and balance. It should *not* be compensation for eating a high-calorie diet. It definitely shouldn't feel like a chore or a punishment. Exercise is like a hobby, something that you *choose* to do, derive satisfaction and pleasure from, want to get better at, and make a priority. You gladly carve out time for hobbies because you love to do them. Exercise should feel like that.

Week One Goal:

Work out the logistics and plan your exercise with a workout buddy.

Make sure that the logistics are easy for both of you because you want this to become a standing date once a week (for now). Every change you make is meant to be integrated into your life easily and slowly. If you move too fast from the get-go, the chances of fizzling out and canceling are high. I want you to be excited and ready for more. If you can work out a second date, great, but don't feel pressure to schedule more than one just yet.

When will you and your workout buddy exercise together?

_____

_____

Week One Cheat Sheet

Circulation

Drink hot lemon water first thing in the morning.

Hunger

Keep a Hunger Diary.
    Choose a hunger visualization image.

Activity

Map your daily routine.
    Identify a time you can add fifteen minutes of non-exercise activity to your routine.
    Track daily steps.

Nutrition

Eat soup for lunch.
    Choose a soup day and make a new recipe.

Prepare snacks for the week while the soup is simmering.

Nutrify your breakfasts and snacks.

General Health

Establish a pre-bedtime no-screen hour.

Choose a regular bedtime fifteen minutes earlier than what you're used to.

Exercise

Schedule one exercise session with your workout buddy.

Week One C.H.A.N.G.E. Chart

Did you C.H.A.N.G.E. this week? Check each box as you complete your steps. Or put a gold star. Or a smile emoji. Whatever you like. It's your path, your chart, your life. Tracking your progress should be a pleasure, not a chore, and should fill you with a sense of accomplishment.

	C	H	A	N	G	E
Monday	_____	_____	_____	_____	_____	_____
Tuesday	_____	_____	_____	_____	_____	_____
Wednesday	_____	_____	_____	_____	_____	_____
Thursday	_____	_____	_____	_____	_____	_____
Friday	_____	_____	_____	_____	_____	_____
Saturday	_____	_____	_____	_____	_____	_____
Sunday	_____	_____	_____	_____	_____	_____

You Are Never So Far Gone That Change Isn't Possible

Royda struggled with diets and weight-loss plans for her whole life, trying one thing and then another, predictably losing weight at first, only to gain it all back, plus a little extra for her trouble. She came to see me after having a baby at forty-three and struggling under the weight of new motherhood. It was a difficult pregnancy with thirty weeks of bed rest. Before that, she was active, kickboxing and going to the gym often. Afterward, she was hit by postpartum blues, sleep deprivation, thirty extra pounds of fat, a closet full of clothes that didn't fit, and self-esteem that was hanging by a thread. Having left her job to become a stay-at-home mom, she felt isolated and ate to relieve stress and fatigue.

"I had no idea what real hunger was," she said. "I never let myself get to that point. One of the first changes I noticed on the Well Path was feeling thirsty. I'd been eating when I should have been drinking water." Royda got in the habit of hydrating, and her nails, skin, and hair responded like watering a plant that had been left too long in the hot sun. "Feeling hydrated gave me energy to start to work out again. I was extra motivated when my friends joined me."

I was one of Royda's workout buddies. We did Zumba in her living room while the baby slept. "I didn't push it or cram stuff in," she said. "I added a strategy here and there, and tried new things, like spinning. I put the baby in the stroller, even in winter, to get out of the house and rack up steps."

Before her vacation, Royda dehydrated her soups and brought them with her. Her family was completely supportive, which surprised her. "I thought they'd push me to eat and drink because it was our vacation, but they were encouraging about the soup and water. For the first time in my life, I came back from vacation without gaining weight."

At her final assessment, Royda lost fifteen pounds of fat and fifteen years off her metabolic age. She texted me a photo of her wearing pre-pregnancy jeans, and it reminded me of my own Path and how good it felt to feel like myself again once I took off the baby weight. "In the past, I always set a goal weight," she said. "But now, what's the point? My goal is to feel great. I just want to continue to feel good and look good."

14

Week Two

By the end of Week One, you may already start to notice positive changes taking place. After a full week of drinking lemon water and eating soup for lunch, your skin should be improved. Your bowel movements should start to become more regular if they weren't before. If you've successfully kept up with regular sleep and wake times, you probably feel better rested, and, therefore, less hungry and moody throughout the day. People might have even commented that you seem happier or more energetic than usual. In only a week, things are changing on the inside, and it shows on the outside.

The theme of this week is adjustment. The changes you're making should become part of your daily routine. This isn't a diet to power through for a month. It's a course of action to change the trajectory of your longer, leaner, happier life. Integrate the activities into your life every day, and you'll benefit forever. So get used to drinking lemon water. It is pretty easy to do, and it works wonders. Get used to tracking your steps/activity and sleep. Keep noticing patterns in your Hunger Diary. The idea isn't to make you obsessed with your health, but to turn these small questions and thoughts into new habits of mindfulness. Before long, when you're sitting for an hour, you'll get up and take a short walk without having to think about it.

This week, your body is going to make the transition from a state of wanting to a state of receiving. There are a lot of sensations that come along with that. As you transition back to a state of balance, you'll notice that a lot has to be undone before your body can start humming along like the incredible machine it is. This is the week where your body hears you send the signals that . . .

Healthy foods are abundant. Your body will stop asking for more calories to fulfill its needs and feel satisfied with your nutrified meals and snacks.

Activity is normalizing and you are no longer sedentary. Your body will adjust by revving up its systems instead of conserving energy.

Circadian rhythms are back in line. Your body won't think winter is summer, won't be compelled to store fat year-round, and will start to relax into a natural sleep pattern.

Circulation is improving, especially in areas that have been sluggish. Your body will respond by increasing blood flow to meet the body's new needs.

C.H.A.N.G.E. Strategies for Week Two

Circulation

Your circulation is a highway. Continuing to stimulate it reminds the body that this flow is the *new* status quo.

Week Two Goal:

Start pranayama breathing. This is one of my favorite wellness practices. Non-yogis might be intimidated by the idea of doing a breathing exercise. But that's all it is. Just breathing, like you already do thousands of times per day, but deeper. When you first wake up, before you get out of bed, you'll spend three minutes pranayama breathing. Turn to page 63 for step-by-step instructions. I also want you to practice muscle contractions as you breathe. Here's how you do it:

One at a time, contract each of the following muscle groups with each breath in; relax the muscles with each breath out. Start with your toes and feet/fingers and hands, then move upward to your calves/forearms, thighs/upper arms, buttocks, abdomen, and finally, face.

The first muscle groups to contract and relax in time with your breath are your toes and feet and fingers and hands. Breathe in while squeezing them, breathe out while relaxing them.

The second muscle groups to contract and relax in time with your second breath are your calves and forearms. Do this by moving your wrists and ankles forward and back with clenched fists.

The third muscle groups are the thighs and upper arms. Contract the biceps by bending your elbows to "make muscles," then straighten your arms to contract your triceps. Tighten and relax your quads, too.

Next breath, contract and relax your buttocks and abdominal muscles. Just clench your abdomen muscles as if someone is about to punch you and you are bearing down to protect yourself. We all know how to squeeze the butt muscles.

Last breath cycle, contract the muscles of your face. Clench your teeth and squeeze your eyes shut.

Repeat this five-breath cycle three times.

This whole process will take only three minutes, not even a nibble out of your morning routine, and you will feel energized from getting oxygen and nutrients throughout your body before you even get out of bed.

Hunger

For the last two weeks you have been developing an awareness of your individual hunger patterns. You have started to recognize that when you feed your body adequate nutrition and calories starting with breakfast, you can better distinguish between false and real hunger, and that the body's signal of "feed me" is one way it tries to eliminate negative feelings like fatigue, stress, anxiety, dehydration, and sadness.

Week Two Goals:

- Keep tracking your hunger. The only way to see patterns is to have enough data, so keep at it.

- Start using your visualization exercise to differentiate between hunger for nutrients and hunger to stop uncomfortable sensations.

Last week I told you to think of a transport vehicle, like an airplane, coming into view any time you were hungry. This week, think of an image that will represent the uncomfortable sensations that bring about false hunger (anger, fatigue, anxiety, boredom, etc.). The image should be something that can fit in the airplane/bus or whatever you chose last week. I tend to stress eat when I'm anxious. My image for those sensations is a little nondescript man, like a Keith Haring outline. When I'm hungry and anxious, I see many men filling up my airplane. I know that if they're in there, my hunger isn't real. Whenever you feel an uncomfortable sensation along with your hunger signal, visualize that airplane filled up with your uncomfortable sensation image.

Emotional Hunger Image:_____

Activity

Over the last two weeks, you've been tracking your inactivity and counting steps. You've gained an invaluable awareness of where, when, and how long you are inactive during the day. Like my patients, you may be shocked by how sedentary you had been. Now is the time to change that.

Week Two Goal:

Implement the fifteen-minute non-exercise activity you identified last week into your routine. If you have an activity monitor, aim to increase your daily number of steps by the number you recorded earlier in a fifteen-minute period of activity. If you do not have one, just shoot for fifteen minutes of activity and implement it every day.

Weekly Steps Average: _____

Nutrition

After a week of having soup for lunch, you should notice increased energy and healthier bowel movements. All of that fiber scrubbing your intestines is clearing the way for better nutrient absorption. The nutrients in the soup are providing a powerful balance of macro- and micronutrients that are benefiting the longevity of the cells you already have, as well as providing the building blocks for new cells. You are growing more vital and balanced with every bowl.

Week Two Goals:

Make one new soup recipe and continue to eat soup for lunch. If the whole serving of two cups is too much for you to finish, eat what feels right and save the rest for later. Some people's stomachs are so messed up from prior eating habits that they are not ready to receive such a high amount of nutrients. As always, pay attention to your body and do what feels right for you.

Prepare your snacks for the week while the soup simmers: 100-calorie bags of corn popped in coconut oil, mixed dried fruit and nuts, or a portable piece of fruit. You should always have healthy snacks on hand.

Start thinking about how to nutrify your dinners. By now, the Four F's—fruit, fat, fiber, and fuel—are on your mind whenever you eat breakfast or have a snack. You're also mindful of AGEs that come from high, dry heat cooking methods like grilling, searing, frying, sautéing, and roasting. Make the same adjustments to dinners that you have at breakfast. Women on the Path have told me that they're eating so well at breakfast and lunch, it feels natural to keep the good food going at dinner. In my house, this is a real challenge with four other palates to feed. It might be for you, too. In this case, start very small and make progressive changes. Perhaps over time, everyone will see how great you look and feel that they will want to jump on the Well Path dinner train, too.

Tips to Nutrify Your Dinners

Here are ten simple suggestions for getting more out of your evening meal:

1. **Eat fewer animal products.** The ultimate goal is to eat only 10 percent of your calories from animal products (dairy, eggs, and meat). Even small steps toward this goal make a big difference. You will not notice trimming one-quarter of your chicken breast off and not eating it. Especially if you replace it with veggies, legumes, or grains.

2. **Eat more vegetables and legumes.** Bring veggies and legumes front and center in your dinner plans. Vegetarian dishes can offer just as much protein as meat-based dishes, and they provide a variety of nutrients that meat doesn't have. Use some of the new foods and combinations you have learned from cooking the soups to make a plate full of veggies, or simply rethink one of your favorite recipes to make it more veggie-centric. This is where you take your new words and start speaking the language.

3. **Shop.** Go to a new store, someplace off the beaten path, and look for a new ingredient you'd like to experiment with. It's easier to break old habits if you are exposed to new things and ideas. If you haven't been to a Whole Foods or an Asian market, now is the time.

4. **Cook something different at home.** Home cooking is preferable to takeout or frozen box meals. But many of us rely on old recipes or supermarket "helpers" that are high in sodium and fat and low in nutrients. One time this week, experiment with a new recipe, something fresh you've never made before. Remember to use low heat,

wet cooking methods to reduce AGEs in food: steaming, boiling, poaching, microwaving, and stewing. Break out the old crockpot if you have one.

5. **Double up.** If you eat dinner out, ask your server for double the veggies in your dish. Pay the extra few dollars for it, if you must. You'll wind up eating less animal protein and carbohydrates and more fiber.

6. **Use your fist.** Remember, a softball-size volume of food will fill your stomach. Measure portions by making a fist. I've found that usually translates to half of a restaurant portion. Great. I can bring home the other half and have it tomorrow.

7. **Eat before you go out.** I often make myself a mini meal before I go out to dinner or to an event with food so I'm not ravenous by the time I actually get to eat and wind up overeating.

8. **Know your go-to meals.** Determine which dishes will reliably fit into your Path. Maybe it's a clean protein like fish or chicken with vegetables or a big, beautiful salad with dressing on the side. It's helpful to have go-to options in mind when you encounter a new menu.

9. **Order off menu.** If I'm at a restaurant that has nothing appealing, I go off menu and ask if they can make something simple for me. Nine times out of ten, they will. It doesn't hurt to ask!

10. **No worries.** If you can't manage a situation, don't stress! It's one meal. Relax, do the best you can, and pat yourself on the back for being mindful.

Soup recipe #4: _____

Snacks? _____

General Health

Last week, you created a no-screen hour before bed, replaced your phone alarm with an old-fashioned alarm clock, and established a reasonable bedtime fifteen minutes earlier than usual. Hopefully you are adapting well to your new routine. It's not easy, but every minute of sleep counts for hormonal balance and cell restoration.

Week Two Goals:

- Move your bedtime earlier by another fifteen minutes. You might need to record your favorite shows and watch them a day later. Who cares? It's worth the sacrifice—plus you save twenty minutes per hour fast-forwarding through commercials. *More* time that you could spend on activities, exercise, or cooking. Who doesn't love that?

- Set a realistic, sustainable wake-up time and try to stick with it every day, even on the weekends.

Set Bedtime: _____

Set Wake Time: _____

Weekly Average Hours of Sleep Per Night (for those who are tracking sleep with a Jawbone or Fitbit): _____

Exercise

I hope you had fun with your exercise buddy last week. Whether you tried a spin class or climbed a wall, you should congratulate yourself just for showing up. Whatever it was, that one session was a huge step forward in fun, fitness, and feeling proud of yourself.

Week Two Goals:

- Start stretching for 10 minutes post-workout. If stretching was included in your workout, add more to get a full 10 minutes. Most classes relegate the stretching to the last three to five minutes of class, which is not enough. You can stretch immediately after you finish exercising or later that night. Flexibility is one of the five components of fitness for a reason. If your fitness is yoga, you're probably getting enough stretching. But it never hurts to do more!

The Importance of Being Flexible

Here are just a few of the benefits of stretching, from the American Council on Exercise:

Decreased muscle stiffness. You want to be able to walk the day after your workout, don't you? A flexible muscle is also less likely to become injured in exercise or other activity.

Decreased joint stiffness. Range of motion is important for post-exercise recovery as well as longevity.

Better posture. For better posture and proper spine alignment, stretch your lower back and chest. Good posture helps you look taller and slimmer!

Less stress. Stretching helps to release tension in your body and your mind.

Improved circulation. Tense muscles slow blood flow; stretching keeps things moving.

Enhanced performance. Supple muscles and joints will allow you to move faster and be stronger.

When will you and your buddy be having fun this week?

Basic Stretching

Here's a brief guide to stretching every major muscle group from Los Angeles–based personal trainer Lalo Fuentes. All you need is 10 minutes and a small spot on a carpeted floor or your yoga mat.

Hamstrings. Sit down on the floor with your legs extended in front of you. Bend one leg so that the bottom of your foot is facing the interior knee of the opposite leg. Sit as tall as you can, then face the foot of your extended leg and lean your torso over as far as you can without pain. Reach your hands toward your toes while your toes are pointed up at all times and the knee of your straight leg is flat on the floor. To increase flexibility, use a yoga strap or a towel around the ball of your foot to assist the stretch. Remember to breathe so your muscles get the oxygen they need to move. Hold this stretch for 20 seconds on each leg.

Groin and inner thigh. Sitting on the floor, place the soles of your feet together with your knees bent and extended out. Move your heels a comfortable distance from your body, and, using your arms, gently push down on your knees to feel the stretch in your inner thighs. Make sure to keep your upper body tall and your neck long during this stretch, as if someone is pulling your head up with a string. You don't have to get your knees all the way to the floor, just do what is comfortable for you. Hold for 20 seconds.

Hips. Lie on your back. Keeping your feet on the floor, bend both knees up into a sit-up position. Place your left ankle over your right knee with your foot flexed. Reach through your legs and pull your right knee toward your torso, keeping your back flat on the floor. You should feel a stretch in your right hip. Hold for 20 seconds and repeat on the other side. You can also do this stretch while sitting on a bench. Cross your legs, placing one ankle on top of the other knee, and with both hands reach down toward the ankle that is on the floor. Make sure to keep your hands on each side of your lowered leg.

Arms. Sitting or standing, face a wall with your arms outstretched. Place your right palm flat on the wall. Keeping the right arm straight, rotate your body away from the arm so that you feel a stretch in the front of your shoulder and all the way down your arm to your wrist. Hold the stretch on each side for 20 seconds.

Chest. While you're standing, flex one arm, making an L shape with your palm open and facing forward. Place that arm against a wall corner. Walk a step forward until you feel a stretch in your chest. Your upper arm should be parallel to the floor at all times. Hold for a count of ten, then switch sides. This stretch is great, especially if you are working on fixing your posture, because it releases your chest muscles, leaving space for your back to pull backward.

Back. While standing, hold on to something in front of you that is stable and chest high with both hands. Lean backward, bend your chin to your chest, and squat slightly with a rounded back. You're going to feel this stretch on both sides of your upper back. Hold this position for 20 seconds, then do a small rotation of your hips to one side and then the other until you feel the stretch on each side of your lower back. Hold for 10 seconds on each side.

Neck. While standing or sitting straight, let your neck tilt to the right side ear to shoulder using its own gravity. Place your right hand on the left side of your head to gently pull the ear toward the shoulder. Breathe deep for 10 to 15 seconds while you feel the stretch. Keeping the hand position, turn your head to look at your armpit and hold for 10 seconds. Still keeping the hand position, rotate your head to look at the sky for 10 seconds. Repeat on the other side.

I am a visual learner, and if you are, too, you can see the demonstration of these stretches on our website.

Week Two Cheat Sheet

Circulation

Drink hot lemon water first thing in the morning.

Do pranayama breathing with muscle contractions in the morning.

Hunger

Keep a Hunger Diary.

Think about hunger visualization images for real and emotional hunger.

Activity

Add fifteen minutes of non-exercise activity to your routine.

Nutrition

Eat soup for lunch.

Make a new soup on your designated day.

Nutrify breakfasts, snacks, and dinners.

General Health

Keep a pre-bed no-screen hour.

Move your set bedtime fifteen minutes earlier.

Set a regular wake time.

Exercise

Do one buddy workout.

Do ten minutes of stretching post-workout or later that night.

Week Two C.H.A.N.G.E. Chart

Maya Angelou once said, "If you don't like something, change it. If you can't change it, change your attitude." Change is a process of continual, micro adjustments. All you have to do is be open to making them.

	C	H	A	N	G	E
Monday	_____	_____	_____	_____	_____	_____
Tuesday	_____	_____	_____	_____	_____	_____
Wednesday	_____	_____	_____	_____	_____	_____
Thursday	_____	_____	_____	_____	_____	_____
Friday	_____	_____	_____	_____	_____	_____
Saturday	_____	_____	_____	_____	_____	_____
Sunday	_____	_____	_____	_____	_____	_____

15.

Week Three

By Week Two, the women in my practice often speak of feeling a seismic shift in their overall health and happiness, like they're finally moving in the right direction. But some of my patients feel a bit frustrated at this early stage: Where's the massive number drop on the scale?

While dieting in the past, women have experienced a honeymoon period. In the first week or two of restrictive eating, they lose a large amount of weight, sometimes up to ten pounds. What they don't realize is that those ten pounds are usually water weight. If you don't give your body adequate nutrition, it goes looking for energy elsewhere. The first place it turns to is the glycogen stores in your muscles and liver. Glycogen, a carb, binds with water molecules. So for every gram of glycogen you "burn," you lose 4 grams of water.

Water weight loss will make you smaller temporarily. It's reassuring emotionally because all of your deprivation and obsessing seems to be paying off. But it's not. Yes, you're losing bloat. You're also losing lean muscle mass. You're *not* losing excess fat. Water weight loss actually ups your body fat percentage, which is the real number to watch for fitness, health, and metabolic age, not a meaningless number on a scale.

Increasing lean muscle mass and decreasing body fat is our goal. Fixing water retention belongs in the circulation category, not here!

So, do not despair about not seeing a dramatic dip on the scale in the early stages of the Path. You are working toward gaining muscle and losing fat, but that beneficial combination of events doesn't show up on the scale just yet. Sometimes it doesn't show up on the scale at all; I've guided women on the Path to zero weight loss. They've lost plenty of pounds of excess *fat* and replaced it pound for pound with lean muscle mass, so they look amazing, have a lower metabolic age, and their clothes fit differently. Weight numbers don't matter. Excess fat matters. How you feel matters. Fitness matters. On the Well Path, you change your mind-set to focus on what matters.

It took me nine months to lose fifty pounds using these strategies, and I have kept it off for five years. I was just like you, busy, stressed, and at the bottom of a mountain that I couldn't see the top of. But now I am stronger than I was in my twenties, with enough energy to make it through the ups and downs of a very hectic life and still do the activities that bring me joy. You can do it, too.

The theme of this week is faith. Have faith that every C.H.A.N.G.E. you are making is bringing you closer to the mountaintop. You are so close to homeostasis! Keep your head down, focus on what matters, and move those feet forward one step at a time.

Cheating

I don't talk about "cheating" with my patients who are on the Well Path because I reject the entire concept. That said, I thought I'd mention it here because it is so ingrained in us to feel shame and guilt for not being perfect in discipline and habit.

Bingeing or "cheating" is a hallmark of Diet Think. On the Well Path, your only goal with food is to nutrify your body on a cellular level. "Good" and "bad" food labeling doesn't exist here, only the mindful choice between nutrient-dense and calorie-dense food. When women say, "I cheated, and then just spiraled down into a major binge," I just want to give them a hug. They beat themselves up for nothing. It's okay to indulge! Good cake is delicious! What would life be like if we couldn't have cake? I feel terrible about the emotional torment they put themselves through. That "I'm a failure" self-talk is what causes binge eating in the first place.

There is no cheating. There is only *choosing*. Choose to have some cake. Choose to enjoy every bite. Once you reach homeostasis, you won't care about cake anymore. If you have it, it'll represent celebration, not failure or cheating. One bite to taste it will be enough, or even more than enough. In the meantime, enjoy food. Enjoy life! Keep that smile on your face, and then go take a walk . . . with a friend . . . in the woods! You are EXACTLY where you are supposed to be.

C.H.A.N.G.E. Strategies for Week Three

Circulation

By drinking your lemon water every day for the last two weeks, you've increased circulation in your GI tract, helped to detox your liver, and have probably freaked out at least once when someone used the last lemon in the fruit bowl. I had one client who didn't like the lemon water routine when she first started but later reported raiding the hotel kitchen in Puerto Rico out of desperation not to miss it.

It is important to drink the lemon water and do the pranayama breathing exercise *consistently* to reap the benefits of a ramped-up circulatory system, which produces more blood flow and oxygenation throughout the day.

Week Three Goal:

Dry brush your body at least once a day. Choose a time during the day when you can integrate dry brushing into your routine.

Traditionalists recommend you do it *before* a shower. The dry brushing sloughs off the dead skin cells, exfoliating your skin. When you follow dry brushing with a shower, all of that gets washed away. But if a pre-shower dry brush isn't possible to integrate into your daily routine, just pick a time that does work. Consistency with dry brushing, like with pranayama breathing and drinking lemon water, is key. The body does not respond to intermittent stimulation in a real way—its fallback position is to conserve energy or stay the same. To effect change, you have to create a new habit. Show your body you mean business with repeated nurturing actions and it will gladly change for you. When will you dry brush every day? Write it down.

The Best Time to Dry Brush Every Day: _____

Dry brushing builds on the previous two weeks of circulation practices. Your body senses a change. It realizes that it needs to increase circulation because of the extra stimulation it's been receiving. Dry brushing amps up that stimulation and takes it to the surface of your skin, expanding and regenerating new healthy blood vessels throughout the body. Dry brushing mobilizes the lymph and the harmful oxidative waste that sits around your cells.

Dry brushing step-by-step:
Brush the soles of your feet from your toes to your heel. Then from your toes on the top of your foot to the ankle. Five to ten light brush strokes are perfect.

Move up your legs, ankle to knee in the front, and ankle to back of the knee in the back. Knee to groin in the front and back of the knee to base of the buttocks in the back, moving the brush in an upward stroke-like motion, always toward the heart.

Buttocks get brushed from the midline bottom nearest your inner thighs toward your saddlebag area, and then up toward your hipbone in a half circle–like motion.

Then brush your trunk below the belly button DOWN toward the groin, and above the belly button UP toward your breasts.

If you have a long-handled brush, do your back next, the whole lovely length of it in an upward motion. Otherwise, make short strokes upward as far as you can reach.

Brush your arms from your fingertips to your elbows and your elbows to your collarbone or armpits.

Brush along your neck down toward your collarbone, your breasts up toward your collarbone, and your shoulders toward your heart center.

For your face, get a softer bristle brush or just use your fingers. Start at the forehead in the middle and brush to the temples, from the midline cheeks to the temples, and the midline around the mouth to the end of your jaw below your ears.

Don't worry about getting every inch of skin. I'd rather you do a poor job of dry brushing seven days a week than a perfectly thorough job twice a week. Consistency is key.

Hunger

By now, you should be much more aware of your hunger patterns than you were before you started the Path. You are also better able to distinguish real hunger from emotional cues. Creating visual cues to represent both types of hunger effectively separated the two sensations in your brain. The more you practice this new awareness, the more your brain will generate new neural pathways that support your new responses. Over time, identifying and responding to real hunger will become second nature.

Week Three Goals:

Keep your Hunger Diary.

Begin to reset your hunger point. Use your imagery to change the way you think about hunger. It sounds complicated, but it's not. If hunger has an uncomfortable feeling associated with it, fill the plane with your visual cue that represents the uncomfortable feeling. If there is no uncomfortable feeling and you are simply ready for food, the plane should come into view empty, but the plane filled with uncomfortable feelings can be acknowledged and sent away to drop off those sensations at another destination. The empty plane can land and you can nourish your body. With the above images in mind, go through the following steps to start resetting your hunger.

Feel the hunger. Remember, hunger is *not* controlled with will-power. It is a basic instinct. Suppressing or ignoring it will only make it speak louder. Visualize the empty plane coming into view.

Register it as real or false. Is the gnawing feeling accompanied by an uncomfortable feeling? If the answer is yes, acknowledge it by filling that plane up with your uncomfortable sensation images. Then let the image fly away. Feel it, don't feed it.

If you're not sure, keep your plane empty and drink a glass of water, wait fifteen minutes, and if it returns repeat steps one to three.

Should it come back *again*, breathe deeply (in for three seconds, out for three seconds), eyes closed, for five consecutive breaths, then repeat steps one to three and wait another fifteen minutes.

If hunger persists for half an hour from your first visualization exercise, have one of your nutritious snacks.

Activity

Last week, you swapped fifteen minutes of tush time for fifteen minutes of non-exercise activity per day. That's a thirty-minute swing toward better circulation and a faster metabolism. You might have achieved this by parking farther from work, or taking more desk breaks to stretch your legs. However you found your fifteen, you deserve a hearty congrats! Along with the activity, you're increasing awareness of how often and for how long you sit during the day. It's enough to make you want to stand up while reading this page. You're probably also feeling the effects of that activity. Women always report better sleep, more overall energy, sharper concentration, and stronger ability to handle stress at this point in the program. You are more likely to stick with your exercise goals on days that you are active as well. And don't forget, activity during the day primes your body to liberate more fat during exercise.

Week Three Goals:

If you're using a fitness monitor, hit your daily steps average from last week *every* day this week.

Identify where you can add your next fifteen minutes of non-exercise activity into your day. Could you walk somewhere instead of driving? Or take a walk during lunch? If you are getting up from your desk three times during the day for five minutes each, could you do it six times instead, or take three ten-minute breaks? Maybe you could walk laps around the parking lot instead of sitting in the car as you wait for your kids to finish soccer practice? Or take an after-dinner stroll, which aids digestion and gives you fresh air before bedtime? You don't have to add the minutes this week. Just identify when you can realistically integrate the next fifteen into your routine.

Daily Steps Average: _____

Where Might You Find Another Fifteen? _____

Nutrition

You've made enormous gains by nutrifying your meals over the last two weeks. You have been eating nutrient-dense soup every day for lunch. You don't have to ask yourself, "What's for lunch today?" because you already know. My patients consistently report that this change relieves their anxiety about making smart lunchtime choices.

You've also been nutrifying your favorite breakfasts and replacing processed food with healthier whole versions. You're developing the "preparation" habit by making your soups and snack bags ahead of time for the week. You've probably noticed that your appetite for late-night snacking is way, *way* down. When you feed the body the nutrients it needs, it doesn't scream for calories at the end of the day.

Continue with the three breakfast choices this week. For the time being, having limited options is helpful. If you feel like it, you can begin experimenting with different ways to nutrify those three favorite breakfasts. Or, you may find comfort in not having too many choices in the beginning while you are mastering your new routine. I promise that in a few weeks, we will add lots more variety.

Week Three Goals:

- Add one more soup to your lineup, bringing your total to five soup varieties to choose from (more if you have a soup buddy).

Soup Recipe #5: _____

- Think of three foods you like and eat regularly that are Calorie Busters. Calorie Busters are foods that can single-handedly slow your fat loss. Some common Calorie Busters are nut butters, butter, cheese, cooking oil, salad dressing, smoothies, ice cream, cookies, mayonnaise, chocolate, honey, syrup, frozen yogurt, hummus, pasta, cereal, and wine.

Nutrient dense, maybe. Calorie dense, *definitely*. Even if the food is healthy, excess is excess. This week, use measuring cups or spoons to assess how much of your Calorie Busters you usually use. You will probably be shocked at how many servings of them you are actually eating and how many calories go along with them. No judgment. Just an exercise to raise awareness. We all have Calorie Busters in our lives. Keep them in your life to prevent feeling deprived, but be aware of their impact on goals.

My Calorie Busters are peanut butter, olive oil, and cereal. I love cereal and it's not leaving my life anytime soon. I have never met a single serving of cereal that seems like it's nearly enough. But I'm aware of my Calorie Busters, and I know that I can be satisfied with half of what I would eat if I were mindlessly pouring. Satisfaction, not deprivation, is key here. I guarantee, when you become aware, you are just as happy with less.

Calorie Buster #1: _____

Calorie Buster #2: _____

Calorie Buster #3: _____

Keeping Things Regular

Nine out of ten women on the Well Path notice immediate, wonderful changes in their digestion and regularity. Occasionally, though, it takes some time to adjust to the increased fiber. My patient Lana, sixty-three, suffered from constipation during her first few weeks on the Path. Before she began the program, she said she was consistently constipated and would regularly use laxatives to move her bowels. I made her stop that regimen immediately and start taking blue-green algae supplements. I also made sure she was drinking her hot lemon water first thing every morning. After a week, her bowel movements started to regulate.

Another patient told me she became constipated anytime she ate beans. I know, we think of beans as being good for elimination—but not for everyone. My prescription for her was drinking an *additional* 20 ounces of water per day, and to hang in there with the soup. I suspected that too many years of not eating enough fiber had slowed her digestion to a crawl—she had to wait for it to regulate itself. Eventually, she became regular and could eat beans and grains and any cruciferous vegetable on the planet without any ill effects.

If you are experiencing some constipation during your first few weeks on the Path, it's likely because your body needs to adjust to processing so much fiber. Make sure you are meeting your hydration goals (half your body weight in ounces of water per day). You can also try adding a tablespoon of extra-virgin olive oil to your lemon water each morning. Klamath Blue Green Algae supplements are a safe alternative to laxatives and stimulants to keep your gut and elimination healthy. It will eventually regulate. Your body needs to adjust, and it will.

General Health

For the last two weeks we've been focusing on sleep. Tracking your patterns makes you conscious of how many hours you actually get (probably not enough). It also helps you notice how your well-being is affected by the amount and the quality of your sleep. Sleep is the cornerstone of physical, mental, and emotional health.

Week Three Goals:

If you're not getting seven hours of sleep per night, move your bedtime earlier by another fifteen minutes.

Set bedtime: _____

Set wake time: _____

- Identify three Small Stressors in your daily life. I'm not talking about Big Stressors, like serious illness or financial straits. I mean the things that, standing on the outside looking in, don't appear to be such a big deal and have no long-term consequences. But from the inside, they throw you into a tizzy.

For example, getting the kids to school on time was one of my Small Stressors. It hijacked my emotions. Feeling rushed, I would get frustrated and angry at my kids and my husband and freak out in traffic. By the time I actually dropped them off, I was all jacked up on cortisol and adrenaline. This went on for years. Then I had an aha moment: for all that stress, I realized there wasn't actually a significant negative consequence if the kids arrived late to school. This worry had absolutely no impact on my life *except* how I was reacting to it. What would be so horrible? Nothing. For twelve years, stress over nothing stole two hours a day from me, my family, my staff, and anyone who got in my way between home and school. What a waste of my valuable time and energy. What a toll that must have taken on my general health. Well, I dropped that inconsequential stressor like a hot potato and my mornings have been totally liberated from that toxic reaction to it.

The consequences of stressing out far exceeded the consequences of being late. I wasn't able to see the obvious truth because in fight-or-flight mode, cortisol blinded me. Awareness and thoughtfulness are not possible when you're freaking out. Our evolutionary physiology is to blame when stress hijacks reason. If it were possible to nip the hijacking in the first place, you could erase the negative consequences (in life and in your hormones) while presenting your higher self to the world around you. Getting emotionally hijacked because I'm worried about being late doesn't teach my kids the value of being prompt, it teaches them a negative way to deal with inconsequential stressors.

This week identify three regularly occurring Small Stressors in your life, where the physical and emotional consequence of the stress itself far outweighs the thing you're freaking out about. Write them down. For now, just think about the everyday stressors that hijack your emotions.

Small Stressor #1:_____

Small Stressor #2:_____

Small Stressor #3:_____

Exercise

I trust your exercise journey so far has been challenging, enlightening, but most of all fun. You have learned what you like about exercise and how quickly you can improve your fitness. If you've hit a little road bump with injury or illness, stay limber by working out around it. For example, if you overworked your legs, focus on your core for a while. You will heal faster if you continue to exercise, as long as you give the injured part a rest.

I hope the lightbulb has turned on and you now realize that staying in the fitness game is the best way to be strong, fit, and balanced for the long haul. Your body is growing younger and will continue to do so as long as you keep exercising and having fun. Your quality of life is directly related to your capacity to move. I think of it this way: vigor or rigor. The choice is obvious.

Week Three Goals:

Stretch for fifteen minutes immediately after a workout or later that night. That's an increase of five minutes of stretching per session. Flexibility is one of the five building block types of exercise (cardio, strength, flexibility, balance, and rest). As you age, it's even more important than cardio or strength. Without flexibility, your body can't recover, gain strength, or be resistant to injury.

Add a second workout to your schedule. Remember, the body responds to repetitive signals. You will build on your skills if you repeat them. If you are running, keep running. If you are cross-training, then cross-train. If you are Zumbaing . . . you get it.

Resting for a day between workouts is crucial to the Path. Going too hard or too frequently is not sustainable and not hormonally fortuitous. Ramping up too quickly has a boomerang effect: It will come back around and knock you off your routine. Go too hard, and you'll use glycogen for energy rather than fat. And then, when you slow down, as you inevitably will, your body will be so confused by the change, it won't regulate your metabolism quickly enough and you'll wind up gaining weight even if you reduce overall calories. If you start slowly and build fitness at a steady pace, your body will stay revved up, use fat for energy, and won't go into a metabolic meltdown if you have to ease off due to injury or life circumstances.

Week Three Cheat Sheet

Circulation

Drink hot lemon water first thing every morning.

Do pranayama breathing when you wake up.

Dry brush every day at the same time.

Hunger

Keep a Hunger Diary.

Practice the visualization exercise when hungry.

Activity

Do thirty minutes of added activity every day.

Mindfully increase daily step average by 10 percent.

Identify when you can add another fifteen minutes of activity to your day and do it.

Nutrition

Make soup and snacks on your usual day.

Eat soup for lunch.

Eat one of your three nutrified breakfast options.

Eat a dinner that's low in AGEs and high in the Four F's.

Identify three Calorie Busters; measure a single serving of each to raise awareness about portion size.

General Health

Keep a no-screen pre-bedtime hour.

If you're not getting seven hours of sleep per night, move your set bedtime fifteen minutes earlier.

Identify three Small Stressors.

Exercise

Do two buddy workouts.

Take a rest day in between workouts.

Stretch for fifteen minutes after each workout or later that night.

Week Three C.H.A.N.G.E. Chart

I love this quote from *Wild* by Cheryl Strayed: "I was amazed that what I need to survive could be carried on my back. And, most surprising of all, that I could carry it." Self-reliance is the most powerful skill you can have. Knowing that all you need is within you fills you with power and esteem. You can do this! You are doing it! Mark your chart with pride.

	C	H	A	N	G	E
Monday	_____	_____	_____	_____	_____	_____
Tuesday	_____	_____	_____	_____	_____	_____
Wednesday	_____	_____	_____	_____	_____	_____
Thursday	_____	_____	_____	_____	_____	_____
Friday	_____	_____	_____	_____	_____	_____
Saturday	_____	_____	_____	_____	_____	_____
Sunday	_____	_____	_____	_____	_____	_____

16

Week Four

By Week Four, most of the women in my practice reach homeostasis. Along with looking great and having more energy, your immune system should now be working on all cylinders. You may notice that you recover from the slightest illness or injury at lightning speed. Colds will last for a few days instead of a couple of weeks. One patient told me that she'd pulled her back out while lifting a heavy bag. She expected the injury to last forever, as it had in the past. But after icing her back and taking an anti-inflammatory for two days, she was better.

Your body wants to be in balance. It wants to heal and be strong. If you provide it with proper rest, nutrition, and movement, it will reward you with radiant health. Why would a cold be dramatically shortened on the Path? Every aspect of it boosts your immune system. Why would a back injury heal so quickly? Strong, supple muscles are in better condition. Your increased circulation zooms healing immune cells through clearer vessels to where they need to go. Think of a house that needs just a little repair to be beautiful versus a run-down shack that would take extreme intervention to be livable. For three weeks, you've been getting your house in order.

The theme of this week on the Path is appreciation. Appreciate every improvement you make as you go along and give it its due. So many diets fixate on the idea of "results," meaning weight loss only. Around Week Three or Four, my patients clue into deeper truths about wellness. Not that fat loss isn't important: You have been and will continue to metabolize fat as you march along the Path. During your daily pranayama breathing, I'd like you to meditate on what results you can appreciate *besides* fat loss. You might realize that balance, resilience, power, energy, and confidence are even more rewarding.

C.H.A.N.G.E. Strategies for Week Four

Circulation

Healthy, youthful cells require oxygen and nutrient-rich blood flowing through unclogged, abundant, far-reaching vessels. On the flip side, every cell in your body generates waste that needs to be carried away so toxic sludge doesn't build up. A wider and faster circulatory highway means stronger cells with longer lives and faster regeneration of dying cells.

Week Four Goals:

Add leg inversions plus deep breathing to your bedtime routine. Putting your legs up the wall is like turning your circulation upside down. All day long, gravity has been pulling at your vessels. So before bed, before being flat for, I hope, seven hours, use gravity to reverse the downward pull of blood into your feet by getting your feet up in the air. The blood will flow down your legs and into your tush, which you've been sitting on for many hours. Combining inversions with deep breathing just helps to push the blood along.

Here's how to practice your leg inversions:

At the end of the day, right before bed, lie on your side on a carpeted surface or on a mat that meets a wall with your bottom toward the wall.

Roll over onto your back, bringing your legs up the wall.

Scoot your bottom toward the wall until they meet.

Your body will be in an L shape, with your back on the floor and your legs up the wall.

Take three deep breaths in and three breaths out. Count for three to six seconds while you inhale, and three to six seconds as you exhale.

Don't worry about muscle contraction at night.

Legs up the wall is meant to be a relaxation posture to calm the body before bed, not a challenging yoga routine.

Hunger

You've kept your last Hunger Diary, so rejoice! By now, you are sick and tired of paying so much attention to every little pang. Good. Change is only possible once you've reached saturation level with your awareness. You used to eat because you were bored or stressed or lonely. Now you know that reacting to uncomfortable sensations with food only makes you more upset and more uncomfortable in the long run. You might not have been able to distinguish between your body's need for nutrition and the need for relief from stress. Now you know that the distinction is easy to make, if you pay attention to your visualization cues. This week, I want you to continue to assess your hunger pangs using your visualization tool. I know you might be tired of this exercise, but you can only integrate true physiological change if you keep repeating behavior over and over. Don't quit. Just one more week, and your hunger point will be reset.

Your Week Four Goal:

- Create an eating schedule. You're probably already on a regular schedule for your three meals and two snacks a day. Just make it semiofficial this week by writing down general time frames. For example: "Lunch: noon to 1:30 p.m." You shouldn't go more than four hours between eating, unless you are just not hungry. Don't eat unless you have physical hunger. Otherwise, you forge neural pathways that reward eating without hunger.

I know many diets tell you to eat every three or four hours no matter what. I disagree. If you're active throughout the day and have a well-nourished body with balanced hormones, your metabolism will not slow down if you go four hours or more without food. Do your thin friends force themselves to eat if they're not hungry? No. They eat when hungry and stop when full.

Everyone is different. We all need to nourish our bodies at different intervals. I need a hearty breakfast and then food every two or three hours from breakfast until bedtime. It's just what my body needs, and I have become aware of that over many years of building my hunger awareness. When my body needs to eat, I must feed it, so I prepare for my eating schedule so that I don't get stuck without something nutritious at the ready.

Eating Schedule

Breakfast: _____

Lunch: _____

Snack #1: _____

Dinner: _____

Snack #2: _____

Activity

By now, you have increased your non-exercise activity by thirty minutes a day, increasing both circulation and fat burn. By adding thirty minutes of activity, you've also subtracted thirty minutes of *in*activity, so your sedentary time has less of a negative impact on your overall health. Only thirty minutes of effort for sixty minutes of benefit!

Week Four Goal:

Balance and increase your activity. This week shift your NEAT movement to happen throughout the day if you are doing fifteen minutes in two distinct blocks. Adding three short bursts (five minutes each) of activity will serve to break up the length of your sedentary stretches. In doing so, you may even find more opportunities to be more active. If you have a fitness tracker, aim to add 10 percent to your step average. Every step you take is one step closer to homeostasis and your goal of looking and feeling like a million bucks.

Weekly Steps Per Day Average:_____

Nutrition

The body wants what the body wants. Your mind might think you crave cupcakes. But your body knows that it'd rather have an apple. After nearly a month on the Path, you have tuned into what your body wants, and know that eating nutrient-dense food makes you feel great, whereas eating sugary, starchy, nutrient-poor food makes you feel bloated and terrible. Your body thanks you, and you should congratulate yourself.

I'm so glad you feel the physical benefits of eating differently without feeling deprived. That doesn't mean you have to refuse every cookie or doughnut that crosses your path. It just means your nutrition has become your priority and you have found a way to make the Four F's yummy and satisfying. Souping, nutrifying, and employing your dining-out strategies have become second nature to you. Keep it up!

Week Four Goal:

Cut your Calorie Busters in half. If you usually spread 2 tablespoons of almond butter on your apples, use just one. If you usually add 2 tablespoons of olive oil to your salad, try using one. If you go out to dinner and normally eat a whole dessert, eat half. You won't miss the other half, I promise. This is not about deprivation, it is about being mindful.

General Health

At this point, I hope you're inching closer to getting a minimum of seven hours of sleep a night. You've also been thinking about the Small Stressors in your life that hijack your physical and mental health. This week, you'll work on resetting your Small Stressor set point and learn

to save your fight-or-flight reaction for the times that are truly worthy
of it.

Week Four Goal:

React to Small Stressors with a verbal mantra. When you feel your nerves
start to fray, say out loud, "There is no real consequence to [insert Small
Stressor here]." You may react or not react, but just keep saying the
mantra over and over. Your friends, kids, and partner might think you've
gone nuts. Let them! They'll be glad if it helps to control a freakout.

Exercise

Whatever you're doing—running, rowing, lifting, hiking, climbing,
Zumbaing—there is no denying the great feeling of regular exercise.
Fitness is exhilaration and joy. It is about strengthening your mind
along with your body, and learning how to face your fears. This week
you will continue your current fitness habit: Exercise with a buddy
twice a week, keep a rest day between workouts, and be sure to stretch
for fifteen minutes on exercise days.

Week Four Goal:

Add a few balance exercises to your routine. You can do these anytime,
while watching TV, just hanging out, or talking on the phone. If your
balance is really limited, use a chair for assistance until you feel confident without one. Lalo Fuentes, a fitness trainer guru, suggested these
exercises to get you started:

Stand on One Leg, Knee Bent
Start with your feet hip-width apart.
Shift your weight to the foot you are going to balance on.
Look at a fixed object in front of you.
Make sure your weight is equally distributed on your standing
    foot (from big toe to pinkie toe to heel), which is rooted to the
    ground.

When you feel strong, lift the other foot off the ground and bend
the knee.

Hold for 30 seconds, aiming to increase time to 1 minute. If you
falter before 30 seconds, just keep repeating until you have
tried to balance for 30 seconds.

Repeat on the other side.

Standing on One Leg, Backward

Start with your feet hip-width apart.

Shift your weight to the foot you are going to balance on.

Look at a fixed object in front of you.

Make sure your weight is equally distributed on your standing foot
(from big toe to pinkie toe to heel), which is rooted to the ground.

When you feel strong, lift the other foot off the ground, reaching
your leg straight behind you, and point your toes.

Stay as upright as possible.

Have a chair nearby if you need it to keep from falling.

Hold for 30 seconds, increasing time to 1 minute. If you falter,
keep trying until the 30 seconds are up.

Repeat on the other side.

Tree Pose

Start in the same way as previous exercises.

When you feel strong, place your opposite foot onto your heel,
shin, or thigh above your knee (never place the foot on your
supporting knee).

Your lifted knee points out to the side.

Focus your eyes on a point in front of you.

You can start out doing this against a wall if need be. Position
yourself so your lifted knee can come into contact with the wall
for balance support.

If you want to challenge yourself, put your palms together in front
of your chest, or raise them in a Y formation over your head.

Once you can hold the pose well for 30 seconds or more, you can advance to gazing toward the sky and then to closing your eyes. Repeat on the other side.

One Leg Reach

Once you feel comfortable standing with one leg off the floor, reach down with your opposite hand and touch the tip of the toe of the leg that you're standing on.

While doing this movement, it is important that your knee is loose, your chest is out, and your shoulder blades are together.

Also, while reaching down, push your hips back. This will make your back straight and put more emphasis on your hamstring/glute area.

Do up to 15 repetitions on each leg.

If the bottom of your foot cramps, stop and do a quick foot stretch before continuing.

Tie Your Shoes

Undo the shoelace of the shoe on the foot you're planning to raise. While holding your balance on one foot, raise the opposite knee (and the foot with the untied shoe) toward your chest.

Keep your ankle flexed while reaching down toward your shoe.

While keeping your balance, tie your shoelace without holding your shoe.

Put down your foot and change sides.

Work up to doing this 10 times on each leg.

For video instruction and more of these balance exercises, you can visit our website.

Continue to be aware of what feels good on your fitness journey. Ultimately, life is an exploration of the whole wide world, and the world inside your own body. Learn what you're capable of. Push your limits. Love the journey.

Week Four Cheat Sheet

Circulation

Drink hot lemon water every morning.

Do pranayama breathing every morning.

Dry brush at the same time each day.

Put your legs up the wall every evening.

Hunger

Use the hunger point reset visualization exercise.

Create an eating schedule.

Activity

Do thirty minutes of additional activity per day.

Add 10 percent to your daily steps average.

Try to make your step graph balanced, with some movement every hour, instead of spiky.

Nutrition

Continue making soup and snacks on your designated day.

Eat soup for lunch.

Eat nutrified breakfasts.

Eat a dinner that's low in AGEs and high in the Four F's.

Cut Calorie Buster portions in half.

General Health

Turn off screens one hour before bedtime.

If you're not getting seven hours of sleep per night, move your set bedtime fifteen minutes earlier.

Be mindful of Small Stressors.

Repeat the mantra to combat Small Stressors every time one comes up.

Exercise

Do two buddy workouts.

Take a rest day in between.

Stretch for fifteen minutes post-workout or later that night.

Do balance exercises once a week.

Week Four C.H.A.N.G.E. Chart

"What you think, you become. What you feel, you attract. What you imagine, you create," said the Buddha. Think, feel, and imagine only the greatest things for yourself. Why not?

	C	H	A	N	G	E
Monday	___	___	___	___	___	___
Tuesday	___	___	___	___	___	___
Wednesday	___	___	___	___	___	___
Thursday	___	___	___	___	___	___
Friday	___	___	___	___	___	___
Saturday	___	___	___	___	___	___
Sunday	___	___	___	___	___	___

Halfway There Questionnaire

When you've finished Week Four, it's time to do another assessment.

What is my body fat percentage? _____ OR How do your jeans fit? Compare photos from Prep Week to this week. Do you notice a difference?

Rate the following from 1 to 5 (1 being the lowest and 5 being the highest):

Energy:_____

Sex drive:_____

Sleep quality: _____

Aches and pains: _____

Bowel movements: _____

Fitness:_____

Mood: _____

Stress coping: _____

Concentration: _____

Memory: _____

17

Week Five

You have made amazing progress in just a matter of weeks, and my guess is that you feel the difference from your bones to your skin. You deserve that spring in your step and the feeling of invincibility. You truly are a Super Woman. That's why the theme of this week is confidence.

You are now confident about expanding your cooking repertoire and about trying new ingredients.

You're confident that your bowels are soaking up nutrients in the food you eat and are moving regularly.

You're confident that your hunger is manageable, and is no longer the enemy.

You're confident that you're growing stronger, leaner, and fitter by the week and that you are physically capable of achieving great things, things you hadn't previously imagined.

You're confident that you have the energy to face the challenges life throws at you, and the wherewithal to manage your stress.

Most important, you have confidence that change is not only possible for you, at this stage of your life, but that it is inevitable if you make the small changes on the Well Path. All you have to do is keep doing what you're doing, and add a few new steps as you go along.

Confidence is the reward for hard work and real life experience. You've earned the right to hold your head up high and say, "I am *killing* it."

C.H.A.N.G.E. Strategies for Week Five

Circulation

In four weeks you have learned how to stimulate your circulation. The obvious improvement in the vibrancy of your skin and eyes and the uptick in your energy level can be directly attributed to your healthy circulation. By now, starting the day without lemon water and deep breathing would seem weird. Good! I want you to feel weird if you don't take advantage of these simple habits that make such a huge difference.

Week Five Goal:

Start to incorporate hot/cold showers at least once a week. I can practically hear the groans. When I first started doing this, I groaned as well.

Remember, the heat causes blood to flow away from your core and rush to your extremities; cold does just the opposite, keeping your vital organs warm. So moving from hot to cold quickly forces your blood to flow out, then rapidly back in. If you pay attention, you can actually feel it happening.

After a little practice, hot/cold showers are an absolute blast. They feel good and boost total body circulation, accelerating and widening your vessels from the tips of your toes to the top of your head in two minutes.

Here's how it works:

Start with your usual warm shower.

Do your cleaning business.

Turn the heat up for thirty seconds and let the hot water wash over you.

Then turn the hot water down to make it cool enough to feel slightly uncomfortable. Let the water wash over you for thirty seconds. Scream, laugh, yell, "I curse you, Dr. Jamé!" Whatever gets you through it.

Those willing can go back to hot for thirty seconds.

Back to cold for thirty seconds.

Get out of the shower.

Take a second to note how you feel.

Hunger

You've visualized, diaried, kept a meal schedule, and reduced your Calorie Busters for four solid weeks. On occasion, you might still be eating out of stress, boredom, anxiety, or thirst, but now you know you're doing it. Being mindful makes all the difference in the world. You are aware of when, why, and what you're eating, and that's truly amazing. Seriously. You know all you need to know to reset your hunger point permanently.

Week Five Goal:

Think about eating-incompatible activities. If you have hunger pangs between scheduled times, feel it but don't feed it. Do the visualization or do an activity that is incompatible with eating, such as taking a shower, washing dishes, folding laundry, going for a walk (but not toward food), light exercise, or stretching. You get my drift. Choose three eating-incompatible activities to have in your pocket when you need them. As always, write it all down:

Eating-Incompatible Activity #1: _____

Eating-Incompatible Activity #2: _____

Eating-Incompatible Activity #3: _____

Activity

After four weeks of being more active, many of my patients tell me they *can't* sit around anymore. That's because the improved flow of nutrients and oxygen to your joints, muscles, brain, and skin just makes you feel good. Sitting doesn't do that. It makes you feel tired.

Week Five Goal:

Replace *another* fifteen minutes of sitting with moving, bringing your total to at least forty-five minutes of additional activity per day. That's a swing of an hour and a half in the right direction, burning an additional 300 calories per day *without breaking a sweat*. It's all about integration. Make movement a habit that, in its absence, just feels wrong. In your schedule, locate where you can grab those fifteen minutes and fold them into your routine. If you have a fitness tracker, add another 10 percent of steps to your day. For example, if your weekly average has been 8,000 steps per day, shoot for 8,800 this week. As with last week, aspire to keep your step graph even, not in a spiky pattern. Take off your fitness tracker during exercise. Those steps don't count for your non-exercise activity totals. And set your smartphone or fitness tracker to alert you at regular intervals to remind you to take a quick walk or even just stand up.

Where can you find another fifteen minutes per day in your routine?

_____

_____

Nutrition

By now you know that I'm not lying to you when I say that eating well makes you crave healthy food. Your body knows a good thing when it digests it. That doesn't mean you won't want a treat or a slice of pizza every now and again. But since you've been eating clean 80 percent of the time or more, your taste for junk has reduced considerably. What a relief it is to be free from compulsive eating, isn't it?

You know the drill by now. On Week Five, you will continue to prepare soups and snacks, eat soups for lunch, and be mindful about your dinners and the strategies for dining out. But you will introduce two new concepts into your nutrition planning this week.

Week Five Goals:

Cut the frequency of eating your Calorie Busters by half. Last week, you cut the quantity of your Calorie Busters. This week, reduce how often you have them. If you have, for example, half a cookie every day, make it every other day this week.

Choose three new breakfasts and three new snacks you haven't been eating thus far, but *only* if you want to. I've mentioned that eating well is like learning a new language. You're proficient in a basic vocabulary. Creating new breakfast options is how you'll start having a conversation. Add three breakfasts to your nutritional arsenal. How will you nutrify old classics? What ingredients have you discovered along the Path that you'd like to experiment with?

No pressure. No rules. Just think creatively and have fun with creating new meal options. There's only one way to break an egg, but a million ways to prepare one. Sautéed spinach in coconut oil with pine nuts and quinoa for breakfast? Why not? Mashed sweet potato with chia seeds, raisins, and pecans? Sprinkle nutritional yeast on your popcorn? Sounds great. It's your life, your meal, your world. Expand it in any direction you choose, and start sharing your recipes with friends or family. Their taste buds will salute you.

If you want some fellow Well Pathers' creative snack and meal ideas, or to share your own culinary concoctions, come visit our website.

New Breakfast Idea #1: _____

New Breakfast Idea #2: _____

New Breakfast Idea #3: _____

New Snack Idea #1: _____

New Snack Idea #2: _____

New Snack Idea #3: _____

General Health

The Four S's of General Health are sleep, sex, stress management, and social life. In the last four weeks, you've been focused on improving sleep habits. Even if you have adapted your schedule and made the necessary adjustments, getting a good night's sleep might continue to be a challenge for you. If you're not yet up to seven hours or are still struggling with insomnia, be patient. Every step in the right direction brings you closer to your goal. Every additional minute is a win.

Sleep Hygiene Reminders

Don't nap. Build your sleep drive so that you'll be tired at your set bedtime.

Get rid of distractions that keep you awake. If something in the bedroom is bright, loud, or anxiety-provoking, move it to another room.

Bed is only for sex and sleep. You have to train your brain to associate it with only those two things. Don't lounge in bed or watch TV in it.

No coffee after 3 p.m.

No alcohol three hours before bed.

If possible, don't exercise for two hours before bed. This can be tough for working women. Try to get in a workout as early in the evening as possible for your sleep quality later.

Week Five Goals:

- Repeat your Small Stressor mantra to the point of it being automatic. Any attempt to change entrenched habits—yes, flying off the handle is a habit—starts with awareness, recognizing a pattern. Then it moves along to making repeated adjustments to retrain your brain. That's what you'll do this week. Say out loud, over and over, "There are no long-term consequences to [insert your Small Stressor here]. The consequence of freaking out is greater than what I'm freaking out about." It'll take a while before the words have an impact on your ability to modify your reaction to stress. Keep hammering the message into your brain. One day it'll work, and you'll breathe easier about the small stuff.

- Identify three Big Stressors that you have no control over. These are things like job stability, financial issues, illness (yours or someone else's), and difficult people you can't avoid. Big Stressors have both short- and long-term consequences. They're major life issues that can really knock you off course.

Eventually, however, you will look back on your Big Stressors with a different perspective. You can't deal with Big Stressors the way you deal with the small ones. There is nothing more stressful than telling yourself not to stress about something that should legitimately concern you. It makes you feel like a failure, as in, "If I were tougher, I'd be able to handle it."

I've been there. I've been through postpartum depression, a horrible divorce, being a single mom, helping a child with a chronic, debilitating illness, and the ups and downs of running my own business during two major economic downturns. I know you can't stop feeling the stress. The best you can do is chip away at it and try to minimize its effects on your body. If you thought about your Big Stressors all at once, you'd be completely overwhelmed by them. I'll ask you to identify only the top three. You don't have to talk about them with others if you don't want to. I find that getting things off my chest and sharing them with someone immediately releases tension. But if you'd rather not talk about them, just write them down.

Big Stressor #1: _____

Big Stressor #2 _____

Big Stressor #3: _____

Exercise

You have been exercising at least twice a week for a while, and it really shows. Build on that to grow your fitness capabilities and shift your metabolism to using *only* fat for fuel. It's happening already, and at a pretty good clip. Since you are losing fat and gaining muscle, your clothes should fit differently now. Your body looks different than it did five weeks ago. Fitness is body changing and life changing. You *can* go farther and jump higher.

Week Five Goal:

Add strength training to the mix. We can all benefit from getting a little stronger. Start with several basic isometric strength moves. Try the following Lalo Fuentes–approved exercises. Once a week, do three repetitions of each one.

Regular plank. Get on your hands and knees, with your hands directly under your shoulders and knees hip-width apart. Turn the tips of your toes in. Lift your knees to come into plank. Lift your hips so your back is flat and your body is suspended in the plank position. OR:

Forearm plank. Lie on the floor, belly down, your arms bent so your hands are next to your shoulders, palms down. Your toes should be hip-width apart. Lift your hips so your back is flat and your body is suspended in the plank position.

Lower abdominal thigh push. Lie on your back with your knees up, feet out so that your calves are parallel to the floor. Place your hands on your thighs close to your knees. Breathe in and bring your knees into your hands. With your hands, resist the movement by pressing against them. You should feel your abdominal wall contracting.

Side plank. Place your right forearm on the floor while lying on your right side. Stack one foot on top of the other. While keeping your elbow directly below your shoulder, raise your hips off the floor. During this move, you should feel your oblique muscles (the muscles on the sides of your waist) doing the work while you stabilize your shoulder muscles by pulling your shoulder blades together.

Build up to hold each exercise for one minute. How long can you do each one this week?

Regular or forearm plank time: _____

Thigh push time: _____

Side plank time: _____

Week Five Cheat Sheet

Circulation

Drink hot lemon water every morning.
Do pranayama breathing every morning.
Dry brush at the same time each day.
Put your legs up the wall every evening.
Take at least one hot/cold shower.

Hunger

Use the hunger point reset visualization exercise.
Create an eating schedule.
Identify eating-incompatible activities.

Activity

Do forty-five minutes of additional activity per day.
Add 10 percent to your daily steps average.
Try to make your step graph balanced, with some movement every hour, instead of spiky.

Nutrition

Continue making soup and snacks on your designated day.

Eat soup for lunch.

Eat nutrified breakfasts.

Eat a dinner that's low in AGEs and high in the Four F's.

Cut Calorie Buster portions in half.

Cut your Calorie Buster frequency in half.

General Health

Turn off screens one hour before bedtime.

If you're not getting seven hours of sleep per night, move your set bedtime fifteen minutes earlier.

Be mindful of Small Stressors.

Repeat the mantra to combat Small Stressors every time one comes up.

Identify three Big Stressors.

Exercise

Do two buddy workouts.

Take a rest day in between.

Stretch for fifteen minutes post-workout or later that night.

Do balance exercises once a week.

Do isometric strength-building moves once a week.

Week Five C.H.A.N.G.E. Chart

Deepak Chopra said, "All great changes are preceded by chaos." If you're experiencing chaos on your Path, have confidence that it will bring amazing changes! You've already made enormous strides in a matter of weeks. Mark each one as the accomplishment it truly is.

	C	H	A	N	G	E
Monday	___	___	___	___	___	___
Tuesday	___	___	___	___	___	___
Wednesday	___	___	___	___	___	___
Thursday	___	___	___	___	___	___
Friday	___	___	___	___	___	___
Saturday	___	___	___	___	___	___
Sunday	___	___	___	___	___	___

Living Inside Your Body

Maisy, sixty, a breast cancer survivor, came to me because she felt disconnected from her body. "My body tried to kill me. I've been scared of my body, afraid to touch my breasts, for a long time," she said. "I want to like my body and feel like a normal person again."

Due to her busy schedule performing on Broadway, Maisy had been eating poorly and drinking *fifteen* diet sodas a day, every day, for decades. "In every photo, I was holding a diet Coke. I didn't know many vegetables existed. How is it I got to be sixty and never ate a chickpea?" Maisy got a fast education about nutrition just by making the soup recipes—and replacing her soda with kombucha. She learned about new ingredients and how to prepare them. "It changed my understanding of food. My mom used to just pile up the plate. I used to think only about quantity. Now I think about quality, and feel much more full with less," she said.

After eight weeks on the Path and her final reconstructive surgery, Maisy is healing. "I have better energy. I had an orgasm—the first one in years.

I'm not separated from my body anymore," she said. "I'm living inside it."
Because of her surgery, Maisy wasn't able to exercise. But, as she says, "I'm
just getting started in my recovery. I needed to take this time and focus on
myself. Now I love Whole Foods! It's my favorite outing. I'm going to shift
from food to fitness now. The pressure to weigh a certain number is gone.
I've been up, I've been down. Now I want to feel strong and healthy."

18

Week Six

Back in high school, I played competitive volleyball. I considered my-self one of the least talented players on the team. Then my coach sat me down and told me, "I know what's holding you back."

"What?" I asked.

"You're making excuses for not practicing harder, to mask your fear of not being good enough to be on this team. If you stopped doing that and went for it, you'd achieve more and see yourself as part of a team of exceptional athletes."

I did often blame the poor effort on minor aches and pains. To his ears, they were excuses for not trying harder. "Excuses are bricks in a wall," he said. "Keep making them, and that wall will be too high to climb over. You have to start taking those bricks down in order to achieve what you are capable of."

Whenever I'm faced with what seems like an insurmountable chal-lenge now, I visualize that brick wall coming down and stepping over it. This little analogy changed my life. Why would you ever want to imprison yourself behind a wall of your own making?

By the time my patients get to Week Six, I often begin to hear ex-cuses. They're so pleased with their success over the past few weeks that they may start to coast a little. When I hear them saying things like, "I was too busy to exercise this week," or "I had to skip soup day because my husband needed me to do something," or "It's too cold outside to do my activity," I tell them the truth: They are walling themselves off from success with all of those excuses.

Learn to recognize an excuse for what it is. But don't stop there. Go deeper and ask yourself, "What am I afraid will happen if I really went for it?" Many of my patients make excuses based on the same fear: failure. What happens if you try your hardest and you still don't achieve your goals? It's a frightening thought for anyone. Sometimes we are so afraid to feel negative emotions that we subconsciously sabotage ourselves.

Fear and excuses are often compounded by a life challenge of some kind. It might be an illness or an injury. It might be a work- or family-related problem. It's easy to dovetail into a backslide when you're dealing with something else that takes up your time and energy. But facing a challenge can also be empowering.

I learned this lesson all too well when I was writing this book and my twelve-year-old son was diagnosed with a chronic, incurable condition that caused him excruciating pain in his feet and toes. As a parent, it was devastating. While my husband and I searched frantically for answers, I tried to help my son deal with the challenge emotionally. I told him that being strong is what would allow him to overcome this, and that adversity really does make you stronger. Being strong doesn't mean he shouldn't feel scared or overwhelmed, it means that he will get better at overcoming fear each time it knocks on his door. And that every time he overcomes fear, he'll be more confident in his ability to do so. We discussed the ways he could proactively care for himself so that he could feel in control of his body and his mind. And because I'd done everything I could to be healthy myself, I was able to support him as best as I could.

When you are supporting your health, you feel stronger and braver, even when things get tough. And they might get very tough. No matter who you are or what you do, life will throw challenges your way. There are times when we all feel overwhelmed and paralyzed by fear. You can choose to be strong and believe you'll get through it, or you can lie down, let it take over, and make excuses for why you've stopped taking care of yourself. Don't allow fear to knock you off the balance you're worked so hard to establish.

The theme of this week is facing challenges. You've already done so much and I'm incredibly proud of you for every step you've taken. In just over a month, you've made yourself stronger and better able to handle obstacles in your path. I've been so inspired by the patients in my practice as they progress. I watch them become more powerful physically and mentally. Being proactive breeds confidence. With newfound energy and fitness, you can face problems head-on. Do not give up, especially when the going gets tough. Let go of the fear of failure. For that matter, let go of the fear of success. Keep moving forward, one step at a time.

Circulation

The improvement in your circulation is one of the main reasons your body has returned to homeostasis. It is crucial to keep your circulation stimulated over your entire life if you want your body to continue to be vital as you age.

Your circulation practices should feel like second nature to you now. Habit, habit, habit. It takes a month to make a habit, and you're entering the sixth week on the Well Path. Maybe you've integrated some of the strategies and are iffy on others? During the next week, embrace and focus on the ones you haven't fully incorporated yet. Remember, it is never too late to start incorporating the C.H.A.N.G.E.s. They're meant to be lifelong habits. If you have incorporated all of the strategies, devote this week to intensifying a couple of them.

Week Six Goals:

Drink hot lemon water at bedtime, too. In the morning, hot lemon water kick-starts your digestion before breakfast. In the evening, it aids in the digestion of your dinner and will help you absorb all of those nutrients.

Increase the time you spend under the cold water in your shower and/or decrease the temperature. Can you stand another twenty seconds under the cold water? Can you do another five degrees colder? Try it. You'll grow to love it.

Losing the Guilt, Increasing the Joy

When hunger resets, it can be a shock to chronic dieters. One patient, Val, told me about her experience eating out with her daughter. "I was halfway done with my plate, and I realized I was full. In the past, I wouldn't have known," she said. "I would have just kept eating until I'd eaten every single bite of the food on my plate. Now I've separated emotion from hunger. I can stop eating, even if others haven't finished their meal, and pack up my leftovers for later. Earlier on the Path, the feeling of triumph over hunger was like, 'Hunger is my bitch.' But now, I don't feel passionately one way or the other. I eat when physically hungry, and stop when full. It's just so damn healthy! I love it."

Stare down your negative emotions about eating. Really look at it. I'm not a psychologist, but feeling the feeling, as opposed to *feeding* the feeling, gets you a lot closer to dealing with the underlying cause. Plus, by not overeating in response, you don't layer the negative emotion with shame and guilt.

Hormones

What? Hormones? Where's Hunger?

Hunger is done. You have focused on it for long enough. H is for Hormones, too, and this week, we're shifting the focus to certain hormones that will help you on your Path. This week, the spotlight is on oxytocin, the hormone of connection to life, love, and joy. Oxytocin reduces fear, and hence reduces the stress hormone cortisol, which, as we know, leads to the accumulation of belly fat. Oxytocin is released after orgasm, while breastfeeding, and whenever you feel joy and love based on human connection.

Week Six Goal:

Increase your connections to boost oxytocin. Think about five people in your life whom you like or love. Visualize them in your mind and meditate on why you like or love them. Engage only positively with those people. No fighting, no yelling. As much as possible, connect physically with those people. Hug, shake hands, link arms, sit close together, touch their shoulder when you talk to them. By using electronics for communicating, we have literally lost touch. Our bodies and souls need it. This touch does not have to be sexual in nature. It could be taking a dance lesson with someone, hugging a friend, massaging your child's back while they do homework. If you can't physically connect with everyone on the list, get on the phone, write a letter, or Skype. Just make that connection however you can.

Who are the five people you'll make an effort to connect with this week?

Person #1: _____

Person #2: _____

Person #3: _____

Person #4: _____

Person #5: _____

Activity

Sometimes fitting in forty-five minutes of activity on top of exercise can be tough. I completely appreciate that. Life is packed, and it's hard to find the time to add whatever non-exercise activity you've chosen. The best way to squeeze it in is to make the activity part of your routine throughout the day. Spreading the activity out, grabbing five minutes every hour for nine hours in a row, might be easier to manage than finding a big chunk or chunks of time. It's also healthier.

Week Six Goal:

Take a long walk. If you're using a Fitbit or a Jawbone tracker, the walk should be 10,000 steps, or approximately four and a half miles. You can do this on the weekend or whenever you can fit it in during the week. The point is to push your limits and prove to yourself that you have built up your endurance and strength in NEAT activity in short bursts, as well as over long periods of time. Depending on your fitness level, a walk of four to five miles will take you anywhere from an hour to two hours. Block out enough time, bring a bottle of water, and go for it. When you are done, reflect on how amazing it feels to have dedicated this time to yourself.

Nutrition

Changing the way you eat has resulted in amazing changes in your body. Even since last week, you might have noticed a big shift. Your body has realized it doesn't need to hold on to excess fat anymore because all of your nutritional needs are being met. An article of clothing that was tight last week might have some wiggle room now. Your bra cup may gap a bit. Bumps and bulges are less noticeable. Losing fat while gaining muscle makes your body tighter, leaner, and healthier.

So don't fix what's been unbroken. Soup on!

Week Six Goal:

Eliminate alcohol. I find that most of my patients have already cut way back on drinking at this point and don't miss it. But if you haven't, now is the time. Alcohol filtering occupies the liver and prevents it from processing fat. A drink also makes you less conscious of your food choices. And talk about a Calorie Buster: A margarita is anywhere from 200 to 500 calories. A glass of red wine is up to 150 calories. A few drinks can really make a difference in your caloric intake. Just for three weeks, abstain from drinking.

Here are some cocktail alternatives that you can substitute when you are out:

Club soda, lime juice, and bitters

Club soda, cucumber, and lime juice

Club soda, basil, cucumber, and bitters

Club soda, ginger, cayenne, and lemon

At home you can try kombucha. Although there is a slight alcohol content, the benefits outweigh this and it is a good alternative.

General Health

This is your busiest C.H.A.N.G.E. category for the week. You'll take on challenges in two different subcategories: stress and (finally!) sex.

Week Six Goal:

Work on counteracting the Big Stressors that you identified last week. This means that you choose to do something that slows down cortisol and adrenaline response when you start to feel stress gaining traction. Just having the choice of doing something versus being passive and inactive is, itself, a tremendous stress relief. Here are a few ideas:

Go for a walk

Exercise

Write in a journal

Call a friend

Do pranayama breathing

Stretch

Chop vegetables

Listen to music

Pick at least two countermeasure strategies and put them in your back pocket. If you are unprepared when the stress hits, you will have a hard time implementing a countermeasure because stress prevents rational thinking. The countermeasure won't change the stressor itself, unfortunately, but it will help to balance the negative effects of stress, helping you think rationally. Stress hormones take fifteen minutes to drain out of your brain. If you can do something positive during that time, you are helping flush them away while you improve your health.

Write down two countermeasure strategies for Big Stressors:

Countermeasure #1: _____

Countermeasure #2: _____

Add one orgasm to your week.

With your body in homeostasis and your hormones in balance, you may have noticed an increase in sex drive. So the timing is just right for this next step. If you currently have none, have one. If you currently have ninety-nine, have one hundred. To clarify, this can be with a partner or alone. You do not need a partner to reap the benefits of orgasm. This should only be a positive practice. If sexual activity causes stress or anxiety for you, have a nonsexual massage instead.

If it's been a while with or without a partner, start with simply getting used to physical intimacy again. Doing the best you can is good enough.

Exercise

Week Six Goal:

Add one more exercise day into your fitness schedule, bringing you to three sessions a week. There is no need to exercise more than three or four times a week to gain fitness or lose fat. This week, shift the tone of your fitness slightly:

Focus one workout session on strengthening muscle. That means either using your own body weight for resistance, or using weights for thirty to forty-five minutes.

Focus one workout session on increasing intensity. Go harder than usual for thirty to forty-five minutes. This is best done with high-intensity intervals evenly spaced throughout your workout. For example: After a five-minute warmup, increase your intensity for two minutes, recover back at low intensity for two to five minutes, and then repeat.

Focus one workout session on building endurance. Whatever you normally do, do it longer. Run longer. Take a longer yoga class. Swim for a longer period of time. My favorite is to take a longer hike or walk. The goal here is to build stamina. How much longer? Start out with 50 percent longer this week. If you run one mile, run one and a half miles. You might run slower, and that's okay because you are working on endurance, not speed.

Don't forget your stretching, balancing, and isometric strength training. I do mine while I watch silly movies with my kids. Sometimes they join in. Modeling healthy behavior for your children is a great gift. Sometimes, they sit on me, giving me more resistance.

Week Six Cheat Sheet

Circulation

Drink hot lemon water twice a day.

Do pranayama breathing every morning.

Dry brush at the same time each day.

Put your legs up the wall every evening.

Take at least one hot/cold shower, with increasing duration and increasing/decreasing temperature.

Hunger/Hormones

Use the hunger point reset visualization exercise.

Create an eating schedule.

Employ eating-incompatible activities when hungry.

Identity five people in your life and connect only positively with them.

Activity

Do forty-five minutes of additional activity per day.

Add 10 percent to your daily steps average.

Try to make your step graph balanced, with some movement every hour, instead of spiky.

Take one long walk of 10,000 steps.

Nutrition

Continue making soup and snacks on your designated day.

Eat soup for lunch.

Eat nutrified breakfasts.

Eat a dinner that's low in AGEs and high in the Four F's.

Cut Calorie Buster portions in half.

Cut Calorie Buster frequency in half.

Eliminate alcohol.

General Health

Turn off screens one hour before bedtime.

If you're not getting seven hours of sleep per night, move your set bedtime fifteen minutes earlier.

Be mindful of Small Stressors.

Repeat the mantra to combat Small Stressors every time one comes up.

Choose and employ two countermeasures for Big Stressors.

Have one more orgasm per week.

Exercise

Do three buddy workouts.

    Take a rest day in between.

    Stretch for fifteen minutes post-workout or later that night.

    Do balance exercises once a week.

    Do isometric strength-building moves once a week.

C.H.A.N.G.E. Chart for Week Six

One of my favorite inspirational quotes is: "If you try, you risk failure. If you don't, you ensure it." Keep trying and risking. It'll be worth it!

	C	H	A	N	G	E
Monday	___	___	___	___	___	___
Tuesday	___	___	___	___	___	___
Wednesday	___	___	___	___	___	___
Thursday	___	___	___	___	___	___
Friday	___	___	___	___	___	___
Saturday	___	___	___	___	___	___
Sunday	___	___	___	___	___	___

A Little C.H.A.N.G.E. Goes a Long Way

Lana's health took a downward spiral following a hysterectomy and a broken ankle that never healed properly. Stress from caring for her mother, who had Alzheimer's, and getting laid off from her job sent her into a spiral of stress-eating and inactivity. She came to see me at the age of sixty-three, weighing 223 pounds. She described herself as "stuck in a rut" of sitting all day at work, not exercising, and eating bagels for breakfast and buffet-style food like ribs and mac and cheese for dinner. "I was tired all the time, and made horrific choices," she said. "I was bloated everywhere, and I kept getting injured doing normal activities because my balance was terrible."

She was trapped in a negative reinforcement loop. The only way out of it was to take small steps, one choice at a time. The first step was to increase her activity level immediately and start nutrifying her body.

Together, we figured out a practical plan for Lana to get to the gym. She had a long list of excuses—from not having the time to not having the right clothes. I became her fitness buddy and made her accountable to exercise once a week on her way home from work. She started making soup to take to work every day. For dinners, she incorporated the Four F's even when she ate out.

That was it. One workout a week. Soup for lunch. Steps during the day and healthy dinners. In one month, Lana lost fifteen pounds, ten of them pure fat. In two months, she lost another six pounds of fat. Her metabolic age dropped ten years.

"Everything feels so much better," she told me at her most recent appointment. "I look better in my clothes, and I'm not hiding in tents anymore. I'm going to the gym twice a week now, and those sessions have become a real highlight of my life. The ankle that has been bothering me for a decade? It's finally strong and doesn't hurt. I wake up happy. It's a complete turnaround in the quality of my life."

19

Week Seven

Charles Darwin once said, "It's not the strongest of the species that survive, nor the most intelligent, but the ones most responsive to change." I'll refine that to say, "For an individual to thrive, she must be responsive to C.H.A.N.G.E." Looking back over the last six weeks, you're probably amazed you're the same person you were when you took your first step on the Path. The cumulative effect of all of your hard work has moved you closer, and closer, and closer to the top of your personal mountain.

The theme of this week is adaptation. Our society is not conducive to good health. Junk food is available at every corner. We drive to get somewhere we could walk to in ten minutes. We sit in front of a computer or a TV in the evening. We live under constant stress, and are often too tired to exercise. To thrive in this world, we have to adapt. The strategies on the Well Path have already helped you to make healthy changes in a hostile environment. You might not be the strongest (although you are getting stronger). You might not be the fastest (who cares?). But you are the master of your destiny, and you deserve a round of applause and a solid pat on the back for your commitment. If you were in my office I would give you a hug and a high five! Patients often tell me at this stage that with all the positive reinforcement from inner and outer improvement, it's only too easy to keep going.

Circulation

I want you to meditate on the glorious flow of oxygen and nutrients around your body and how well it has served you these past six weeks. If you have integrated some of the circulation strategies, but not others, work on the weaker practices this week while keeping up with the solid ones.

Week Seven Goals:

Pranayama breathing exercise at bedtime, too. Add one more session of deep breathing with muscle contraction as the last thing you do at night before sleep. Just as it serves to wake you up at wake time, it will also help relax you at nighttime.

Dry brush twice a day. A little of a good thing is good. A lot of a good thing is great. If you usually dry brush in the morning when you brush your teeth, add another session of skin brushing when you brush your teeth at night.

Hormones

Last week, you started stimulating the flow of oxytocin by connecting to life, love, and emotional and physical joy. Anything that makes you feel closer to the important people in your life boosts the flow of the "love" hormone. You were tasked with showing your loved ones with words and touch how you feel. Keep it up to maintain or increase the level of physical and connective intimacy with five people you love. Maybe they'll jump onboard and start spreading the love to the people in their world, too.

Oxytocin and cortisol are on a seesaw in your body. One goes up, the other goes down. The oxytocin boost will make cortisol decrease. This week, tip the hormonal seesaw overwhelmingly in your favor.

Week Seven Goal:

Have five daily positive interactions with strangers, acquaintances, or coworkers.

Practice being relentlessly positive in benign situations.

Go beyond saying "please" and "thank you" to cashiers and shop people. Look them in the eye and make it really count. This might feel uncomfortable at first. I admit I used to avoid strangers' eyes. I preferred to fly under the radar and save my conversational energy for people I cared about. But I've found that if you open your heart and make eye contact with everyone, you gain positive energy from it. No one is judging you. I promise, if you say a heartfelt "hello, how are you today?" and give a smile to the cashier at Rite Aid, she will appreciate it and return the good vibe to you or to someone else who might need it. Think of the awesome domino effect you just started.

I call engaging with strangers and acquaintances "stepping up" into humanity. Instead of shrinking back out of fear or insecurity, take that step forward and trust that people will respond positively to you. It allows you to feel the extent of your own power and instantly disarms the person you are "stepping up" to. With every friendly "I see you" gesture, your cortisol instantly goes down.

Activity

If you're using a fitness tracker, I'm sure you've become addicted to increasing your daily steps and using those inactivity alerts to remind you to stand up when you've been sitting for too long. If you're not using a tracker, keep pushing for those forty-five minutes of additional activity and spreading them out over the course of the day. You have probably become so aware of your activity that you can predict where your steps will land. This awareness is all you need to keep this level of activity going, fitness tracker or not.

Week Seven Goal:

Take your non-exercise activity up a notch and add yet another fifteen minutes to replace sitting time. You've spent six weeks building to this point. When you are moving an extra hour every day, you are affecting a *two-hour swing in the right direction*. At this point, you have increased your daily metabolic burn by as much as 400-plus calories. Your body has revved up to burn through an additional 2,800 calories a week, just by being more active. You've bought yourself nearly a pound of fat loss per week, *without breaking a sweat*. Try to use these fifteen minutes to keep yourself from sitting for more than one and a half hours at a time. That is, every one and a half hours, get up and move for a couple of minutes before sitting down again.

Where will you find another fifteen minutes?: _____

Nutrition

Your body is now used to existing in a highly nutrified state. Undoubtedly, you've had days or meals when you didn't eat nutritious food, and your body let you know it wasn't happy about it by giving you indigestion, bloating, carb cravings, a sugar headache, constipation, or fatigue. You have internalized in the most literal sense how good it feels to give your cells exactly what they want.

Week Seven Goal:

Micromanage the timing of your nutrition before and after exercise so you burn more fat and build more muscle. This new habit will ensure you have adequate fuel to push through your extra workout (and to increase your exertion), and will also help you recover, allowing muscle growth and repair to take place. You can't work hard without the proper fuel, and nothing derails fitness like feeling too tired to do it.

Eat More to Lose More

Alake claimed that she was working out five days a week but unable to get more fit or lose weight. She said she was doing her best in her exercise classes but often felt she didn't have the energy to get out of them what she wanted. So we looked at her plan, went over her fitness, and talked about the need for rest. She was doing everything right. Then we talked about nutrition, and a lightbulb went on. We realized that she hadn't been feeding herself properly before and after her workouts. When she started micromanaging her nutrition to coincide with her fitness, she finally understood what it felt like to really work hard in a class and have the stamina for the duration. In her own words: "Now I'm able to do all the moves with oomph! I can finally see results." It was a breakthrough. Her fat loss and muscle gain accelerated from that point on. She had to eat strategically to fuel her fitness gains.

Here's how to time your food with your fitness:

Up to one hour before your workout starts: Have a 100-calorie snack that's half carbohydrate and half protein: half an apple and a hard-boiled egg, half a banana and a spoonful of peanut butter, some nuts and dried fruit, half an energy bar (make sure it's not a candy bar in disguise); even a scoop of protein powder mixed with water in a shaker is a great choice (my favorite brand is Vega One).

Between twenty and sixty minutes after your workout: Have a 100- to 300-calorie snack of half protein and half carbohydrate. Personally, I like liquids post-workout. They are easy to digest and therefore get to your muscles quicker. Protein shakes from the gym or premixed cans can have too many hidden ingredients and are inappropriately calorie dense for the average exerciser—make your own healthy shakes at home, or share a smoothie with your workout partner instead of having one each (half the calories AND half the cost). If you are eating a meal within that time frame, just make sure you include carbohydrates. You must replenish the glycogen in your muscles for fitness sustainability.

Come up with a few pre- and post-workout snack ideas and prepare them ahead of time so you can just grab and go.

Pre-workout Snack Idea #1: _____

Pre-workout Snack Idea #2: _____

Pre-workout Snack Idea #3: _____

Post-workout Snack Idea #1: _____

Post-workout Snack Idea #2: _____

Post-workout Snack Idea #3: _____

General Health

Week Seven Goals:

- Try cognitive behavioral therapy to combat insomnia. One good CBT-based strategy for dealing with insomnia is, ironically, getting out of bed. If you are lying in bed, not sleeping, for fifteen minutes, don't stay in bed. Get up and do a calming activity like meditating or deep breathing for ten minutes. Then go back to bed and try to fall asleep again. Repeat as necessary. It's designed to reduce the anxiety of insomnia, breaking the wake-worry cycle.

- Think about two new countermeasures to Big Stressors this week. Have you found a Big Stressor countermeasure that seems to take the edge off your anxiety? It could be gardening, calling a friend, hugging your child, chopping veggies for soup, or listening to music. By trial and error, keep searching until you find a couple of countermeasures that work well and that you can use whenever you feel stress coming on. The goal is to reduce the rush of adrenaline and cortisol. Countermeasures won't solve the stressor, but if the stressor is solvable, you can't attempt to sort it out with cortisol or adrenaline hijacking your brain. You need a calm mind and body to get through the crisis. Remember, it takes fifteen minutes for these hormones to cycle through. Your countermeasure should last at least that long.

Countermeasure #1: _____

Countermeasure #2: _____

Add one more orgasm to your week. Good thing you didn't start adding orgasms from Week One—you'd have no time to go to the gym by now! If you started with nonsexual touch or gentle nonorgasmic physical intimacy, keep practicing that until you are feeling the urge to take more steps forward. No pressure, just reassurance that you are on the path that is right for you. Don't ignore or give up on your sexual health; it is called sexual HEALTH for a reason . . . it is good for you.

Count your social encounters. The last of the Four S's of General Health is socializing. Guess what? The Path has been designed to increase interactions with people from Week One. Your fitness buddy workouts have added heart- and hormone-healthy interactions to your week. You've been cooking more at home to enjoy dinners as a family. You've been asked to engage with loved ones and strangers every day. Then there's the added orgasms, which you might be enjoying with a partner. Socializing is the connective tissue that runs through the length of the Path. I hope that, as you look back on this experience, you see that you are healthier, more involved in your world, have met new, wonderful people, are closer to people already in your life, and are less afraid to meet new people.

Number of social encounters: _____

Exercise

Week Seven Goals:

Add a fourth workout (optional). Four workouts are more than enough! More than four days of exercise isn't sustainable for most of us, and it's not necessary to reach your fitness goals unless you are a professional or an amateur athlete training for competition (and if you are, make sure you are eating adequate calories to maintain your strength). If your intention is to lose fat, exercising more than four days a week won't make a difference. Enjoy your rest days and let the benefits of your fitness take root.

Increase intensity overall. For all of your workouts, try to raise your heart rate slightly for longer periods of time. See how long you can go. Finding your edge can build self-esteem. Even if it is just one stride farther than last week, you've increased endurance and stamina.

Week Seven Cheat Sheet

Circulation

Drink hot lemon water twice a day.

Do pranayama breathing twice a day.

Dry brush twice a day.

Put your legs up the wall every evening.

Take at least one hot/cold shower, with increasing duration and increasing/decreasing temperature.

Hunger/Hormones

Use the hunger point reset visualization exercise.

Create an eating schedule.

Employ eating-incompatible activities when hungry.

Connect positively with five loved ones per day to boost oxytocin.

Connect with five strangers or acquaintances per day to lower cortisol.

Activity

Do one hour of additional activity per day.

Add 10 percent to your daily steps average.

Try to make your step graph balanced, with some movement every hour, instead of spiky.

Take one long walk of 10,000 steps.

Nutrition

Continue making soup and snacks on your designated day.

Eat soup for lunch.

Eat nutrified breakfasts.

Eat a dinner that's low in AGEs and high in the Four F's.

Cut Calorie Buster portions in half.

Cut Calorie Buster frequency in half.

Eliminate alcohol.

Micromanage the timing of your pre- and post-workout snacks or meals.

General Health

Turn off screens one hour before bedtime.

If you're not getting seven hours of sleep per night, move your set bedtime fifteen minutes earlier.

Be mindful of Small Stressors.

Repeat the mantra to combat Small Stressors every time one comes up.

Employ countermeasures for Big Stressors.

Have two more orgasms per week.

Count social encounters.

Exercise

Do three or four buddy workouts.

Increase intensity overall.

Take a rest day in between.

Stretch for fifteen minutes post-workout or later that night.

Do balance exercises once a week.

Do isometric strength-building moves once a week.

Week Seven C.H.A.N.G.E. Chart

Life is like a roller coaster. Either you can freak out every time you hit a bump or you can scream at the top of your lungs, throw your hands up, and enjoy the ride. Ladies: Hands UP! Voices UP! Let it all out.

	C	H	A	N	G	E
Monday	_____	_____	_____	_____	_____	____
Tuesday	_____	_____	_____	_____	_____	____
Wednesday	_____	_____	_____	_____	_____	____
Thursday	_____	_____	_____	_____	_____	____
Friday	_____	_____	_____	_____	_____	____
Saturday	_____	_____	_____	_____	_____	____
Sunday	_____	_____	_____	_____	_____	____

20

Week Eight

Here we are at Week Eight. For seven weeks, you've been changing and growing healthier and younger from the inside out. You are only a few steps away from your mountaintop.

The theme of this week is internalization. You have everything you need already. It's just a matter of repetition and practice to make sure it's all deeply ingrained in your routine. Focus your efforts this week on internalizing any strategy that still feels like hard work. Even if there was something that you haven't tried yet, you can still start it this week, or anytime. The Well Path doesn't just abruptly end after Week Eight. It keeps going. Anytime is a good time to integrate any part of the Path.

For my patients, Week Eight is like taking a victory lap. I hope it feels that way for you, too. You deserve to celebrate the triumph of wellness.

Circulation

Warning: You are about to face the toughest challenge so far to increase blood and lymph movement in your body. Brace yourself. It's a toughie.

Week Eight Goal:

Get a massage. Mandatory. Go to a spa or to a Massage Envy and treat yourself to an hour-long massage. Not only will it get your fluids flowing, it will increase oxytocin and reduce cortisol in the most relaxing way. Consider incorporating a monthly or bimonthly massage into your routine. Set it on your calendar to pamper yourself, reward yourself, and get the special attention of a professional to reward your body for stepping up to the plate and swinging for the stands.

Hunger/Hormones

Hunger, mindfulness, fueling, and nutrifying have become positively reinforced by now. Why would you do anything else?

Week Eight Goals:

- Revisit your hunger awareness practices. Although you have been doing them all along, give them particular acknowledgment this week, especially during anxious times. By integrating the hunger strategies, you have eliminated a huge source of anxiety and stress from your life. Now you can save those emotions, and the hormonal flow they cause, for when you actually need them.

- Add five positive social encounters with people you *don't* like. Along with your connecting with loved ones and having five positive interactions with strangers and acquaintances you like, I challenge you to extend it to people whom you actively avoid and don't care for. It can be brief, if only a few seconds long. Look them in the eye and smile. If they complain or criticize, interject a compliment or positive observation into the conversation. Who knows what curmudgeon you might soften up and bring over to the bright side of life?

- Connect to a cause. You might not have extra time to volunteer, and you might not know how to go about it if you did have time. All I ask is that you think of two causes that have deep meaning to you—animal rescue, literacy, poverty relief, a political party, community gardening, children. Just think about something you can get behind and support to make this a better world. Don't go deeper than that yet, unless you are motivated to go online to find a particular organization or to ask your friends for suggestions. Start with "what." The "how" will come later.

It is important to have something that you can dedicate yourself to over the years and feel a sense of community and contribution. Thinking of others less fortunate than you gives you the gift of perspective. I've always wanted to join Doctors Without Borders, but that's not possible for me right now with small kids at home. Then I got an idea. One day while hiking, I realized how grateful I was to be able to challenge myself physically in the ability to hike long distances on the Appalachian Trail with my husband. I would be devastated if I couldn't go hiking. My thoughts turned to the people who can't, especially children who have lost limbs.

I researched organizations that provided impoverished children with prosthetic limbs and found A Leg To Stand On. I don't have a lot of time or money to dedicate to this charity, but I do what I can to support them. My husband and I raise funds and awareness by lining up sponsors before we go on our hikes. The farther we go, the more money we raise.

Coincidentally, while raising money and hiking for ALTSO, we came across some military veterans "hiking off the war," as they put it. I was reminded of my days working at a VA hospital, and the profound gratitude I feel toward the men and women who serve our country. Now my husband and I split our dedication between the kids and the vets. Anytime I have an ache or go through difficult times, I think of ALTSO kids and our nation's heroes and gain plenty of perspective. Dedicating your ability and passion to someone or something worthy of them is a grand benefit for you. It doesn't have to be big. It only has to come from the heart.

A Cause You Believe In #1: _____

A Cause You Believe In #2: _____

Activity

By now, sitting for long periods of time makes you feel strange. It might even make your hips and knees ache to be inactive for an hour or two. This is good news! It's your joints and muscles telling you that they need fresh oxygen. Your activity is so well balanced that you've come to crave your five-minute stretch or walk around the block.

Week Eight Goal:

Increase step totals by an additional 10 percent, or swap out another fifteen minutes of inactive time for active time per day. Reminder: Standing counts. Standing up when you're on the phone or during TV commercials will buy you the last extra bit of activity to put you over the top. If you meet this challenge, you will have increased your active time by seventy-five minutes per day, a 150-minute swing in the right direction. By the end of the week, you'll have made a positive change of 1,050 minutes, or seventeen and a half hours, in one week. That's an incredible accomplishment.

Nutrition

Do it all, as you've grown accustomed. Enjoy soup for lunch every day. Nutrify the heck out of breakfasts, dinners, and snacks. Micromanage your pre- and post-workout snacks to maximize your fat metabolism, recovery, and preparation for next time.

In my practice, I've collected soup recipes from patients and have fallen in love with many of them. You'll find them in the recipes starting on page 249. Now it's your turn.

Week Eight Goal:

Create a soup recipe of your own. Remember all the things you learned about the various nutrient combinations you've been preparing. If you need help, go to this amazing nutrition data website and plug in your ingredients to see how balanced they are: www.nutritiondata.self.com.

Name your soup recipe: _____

Submit your recipe through our website and we will cook it up and share the recipe with others.

General Health

Your General Health is paramount to your well-being as well as your ability to regenerate cells and metabolize fat. This week you deserve to focus on the categories that bring you pleasure and joy.

Week Eight Goals:

Get seven hours of sleep at least four nights. Thus far, I haven't asked you to get all seven hours on any number of given nights. But this week, make a point of prioritizing mentally and physically restorative rest.

Have at least three orgasms. It doesn't matter if they're with a partner or by yourself.

Add one more special social encounter. Pay it forward. Use your success to inspire a friend or family member who you think would benefit from being on the Well Path. Offer to be their buddy to get them started. Make a date with them to cook their first round of soup. Now that you are the expert in life C.H.A.N.G.E., you can be a model for how far you can go if you just take one step at a time. Inspiring others is just about the best thing for sustaining your journey and fueling all of those good hormones that keep you young and vital throughout your lifetime.

Exercise

Look back to where you were when you started the Path. Regarding your fitness—strength, flexibility, and endurance—you have improved by leaps, bounds, and planks! You have set and met my challenges week after week. So, during this final week on the Path, I'd like to challenge you to . . .

Week Eight Goals:

Challenge yourself!

 Run faster than you have run before.

 Jump higher than you have jumped before.

 Row faster than you have rowed before.

 Do twenty more sit-ups than you have done before.

 Hold a plank for the longest amount of time ever.

 Most important, reflect on how far you have come since the very first week you started. Know that there is nothing you can't do.

Week Eight Cheat Sheet

Circulation

Drink hot lemon water twice a day.

 Do pranayama breathing twice a day.

 Dry brush twice a day.

 Put your legs up the wall every evening.

 Take at least one hot/cold shower, with increasing duration and increasing/decreasing temperature.

 Get a monthly or bimonthly massage.

Hunger/Hormones

Use the hunger point reset visualization exercise.

 Create an eating schedule.

 Employ eating-incompatible activities when hungry.

 Connect positively with five loved ones per day to boost oxytocin.

 Connect with five strangers or acquaintances per day to lower cortisol.

 Have positive encounters with people you *don't* like.

 Think of two causes you can see yourself joining.

Activity

Do one hour and fifteen minutes of additional activity per day.

Add 10 percent to your daily steps average.

Try to make your step graph balanced, with some movement every hour, instead of spiky.

Take one long walk of 10,000 steps.

Nutrition

Continue making soup and snacks on your designated day.

Eat soup for lunch.

Eat nutrified breakfasts.

Eat a dinner that's low in AGEs and high in the Four F's.

Cut Calorie Buster portions in half.

Cut Calorie Buster frequency in half.

Eliminate alcohol.

Micromanage the timing of your pre- and post-workout snacks or meals.

Create your own soup recipe; send it to our website.

Have a drink! You deserve it.

General Health

Turn off screens one hour before bedtime.

Prioritize getting seven hours of sleep four nights this week.

Be mindful of Small Stressors.

Repeat the mantra to combat Small Stressors every time one comes up.

Employ countermeasures for Big Stressors.

Have three more orgasms per week.

Inspire one person to get on the Well Path.

Exercise

Do three or four buddy workouts.

Increase intensity overall.

Take a rest day in between.

Stretch for fifteen minutes post-workout or later that night.

Do balance exercises once a week.

Do isometric strength-building moves once a week.

Create a personal challenge for yourself, and do it!

Week Eight C.H.A.N.G.E. Chart

Success isn't about how much money you make. It's about making a difference in people's lives. That is my goal, and I hope I've helped you make improvements in your life and the lives of others. Always aspire to make the world a better place.

	C	H	A	N	G	E
Monday	____	____	____	____	____	____
Tuesday	____	____	____	____	____	____
Wednesday	____	____	____	____	____	____
Thursday	____	____	____	____	____	____
Friday	____	____	____	____	____	____
Saturday	____	____	____	____	____	____
Sunday	____	____	____	____	____	____

Final Questionnaire

When you've finished Week Eight, take the final assessment.

What is my body fat percentage? _____

OR How do your jeans fit?   _____

Compare photos from Prep Week, to Week Four, to this week. Do you notice a difference? _____

Rate the following from 1 to 5 (1 being the lowest and 5 being the highest):

Energy:_____

Sex drive:_____

Sleep quality: _____

Aches and pains: _____

Bowel movements: _____

Fitness:_____

Mood: _____

Stress coping: _____

Concentration: _____

Memory: _____

As you can see, the results of the Well Path are more far-reaching than just your weight. Enjoy every benefit that you've worked so hard to achieve!

21

Life in Balance

Congrats! You've completed eight weeks on the Well Path and transformed your health and appearance along the way.

After completing eight weeks on the Path, the majority of my patients reach homeostasis. In fact, most make it by Week Four or Five. How do you know when you've arrived? Well, you could do a long series of blood tests and body scans. Or you could just look in the mirror. Are the bags under your eyes smaller? Is your skin bouncier and smoother, less red and spotty? Are the whites of your eyes brighter? Or just look into your intuition. Do you have the sense that everything feels "right"? It's an amorphous measurement, but it can be meaningful.

In my practice, I use this Homeostasis Checklist:

☐ Do you fall asleep within fifteen minutes of going to bed and stay asleep until morning?

☐ Are your bowel movements regular and the consistency of toothpaste?

☐ Do you have fewer aches and pains than a month ago?

☐ Is your energy level increased?

☐ Has your sex drive improved?

☐ Have you stopped craving sugar or junk food?

☐ Do you feel fuller by eating less food?

☐ Has your concentration improved?

☐ Are you stronger?

☐ Is it noticeably easier to walk up stairs?

If you answered "no" to three or more of these questions, you're not quite there yet. Keep up with the strategies, and revisit this checklist in a week. Those who marked "yes" to at least seven of the ten questions, you've made it! Now that you're in balance, your body can do what it was designed to do—metabolize fat for energy, regenerate and repair cells rapidly, and react appropriately to external and internal hormonal cues. Now that your body is no longer in survival shutdown or fight-or-flight mode, you can *thrive*. The pace picks up now because your body is like a well-oiled machine that wants to run and shout with joy. After eight weeks of making changes, you have reached your goal.

Now what?

Keep going! Repeat your Week Eight victory lap over and over again. Modify your Path as you see fit. It's yours to play with, fine-tune, and enjoy for the rest of your fit, fabulous life.

But what would happen, say, if your life changed and you slipped off the Path? Circumstances aren't always constant. During our winter session last year, one woman in the program had to move. Another had to travel extensively. Another woman lost her job. Another got pregnant. Another got the flu.

Life does not exist in a vacuum. The Well Path has a lot of wiggle room to accommodate upheavals big and small. When circumstances change and throw you off your established routine, don't panic. Just do the best you can. You might not be able to do it all. But if you can check a few items off your list, you're taking steps in the right direction. If you can't cook, make the most nutritious choices you can with the options available. If you can't exercise, try to be as active as possible throughout the day. If you can't have sex, explore alternative ways to relax. Try to squeeze in ten minutes of stretching on the floor. Do vinyasas in the living room if you can't get to yoga class. The more you can do, even if it's only for five minutes here and there, the better you'll feel.

The worst thing to do is to write off the Path until crunch time is over. It is better to stay on it in any capacity than to throw the strategies out the window. Even if you only have hot lemon water before breakfast, you're still starting the day mindful of your health. Walking for five minutes every hour will help you concentrate at the new job, recover from a cold or injury, thrive under pressure, and be a happier, more energized person for those who need you.

A complete regression back to your previous "unhealthy" habits is, obviously, a giant step backward. I've noticed that some women, at the slightest fluctuation in weight, say or think, "I'll just cut out carbs for a week or two."

Please, please, please don't revert to the destructive habits that caused nothing but frustration, guilt, blame, and shame—not to mention weight gain. If you feel tempted by old bad habits, just be aware that you've been there, done that. You know how to fail. Instead, practice success. Practice facing your fears. Acknowledge that perfection is a myth.

Use visualization with your bad habits, like you did with hunger. See the habit or unhealthy desire fly into your consciousness. Acknowledge it, study it, detach emotionally from it, and then let it fly away. When I notice old habits turning up, I throw a bunch of Well Path strategies at them. I have some hot lemon water or do pranayama breathing. I take a walk or call a friend. I know the bad habit will circle in and out of my mind for a few days, especially when I'm stressed or tired. But I keep doing countermeasures and it flies away—until the next time. The solution is to rationally, logically decide to do what you know will make you feel better, and not give in to the self-destructive desire to do what you know will make you feel terrible.

If, for whatever reason, you do veer off the Path, it's okay. Just gently, slowly consult your GPS (this book) and find your way back. As you progress, think BIG. Diets are small. They're about putting yourself in a tiny box. On the Well Path, the world is at your feet. Go anywhere, do anything. Always remember the values you've been learning along the way.

It's all about you. The Well Path is individual. You choose your own foods and fitness. You become the expert of yourself. You are in tune with your body like never before. You know what hunger feels like. You know that your ability to change is limitless. Bring all that expertise to everything you do.

Success is when you start. Take that first step, and it's like you're halfway there. Why? One step leads to the next. One step after another is the formula for climbing your mountain, no matter how high.

Keep moving forward. If you're standing in the middle of a tightrope, you can move forward or backward with the same risk. So you might as well move forward. With each step forward, ask yourself, "Why am I on the Well Path? What do I hope to achieve? What is at stake? What makes me feel good about myself? What makes me feel bad?" Your feet will take care of the rest.

Don't go in circles. We can all get complacent. We phone in our fitness and stop pushing our limits. Your life and your health deserve your full effort. Without them, you've got nothing.

Appreciate where you've been. I always ask my patients to remind themselves what their life was like before they took their first tentative steps on the Path. The difference is incredible. To stay on the Path, look at how far you've come. Drink in that perspective and be proud of yourself.

If it's not sustainable, it won't work. Don't push yourself so hard or so far that you can't maintain what you're doing. Organize your strategies into your life in a way that is doable.

Change doesn't have to hurt. A lot of my patients can't believe they got to the end of the Well Path so easily. Apparently, they thought they'd be crawling to the mountaintop with bloodied knees and sunken eyes. But they leapt to the summit and took a million smiling selfies. While enjoying the view, they appreciated how far they'd come and how much they'd accomplished—and it wasn't hard at all.

Pat yourself on the back. Women don't cheer themselves on enough. We need to say, "I'm great! I rule! I'm awesome." Make it a mantra. "I'm a badass. I'm stronger than I thought. I mean business." Negative self-talk must be banished.

Share yourself! You are part of a family, community, and world that needs healing and love. Transform your outlook by taking someone's hand. Reach out to a friend. Bring others with you on the Path. Be the person who smiles at the scowling employee behind the counter. Share kindness.

Integration is everything. Your C.H.A.N.G.E.s should be automatic, a part of your day, as second nature as brushing your teeth and turning off the light before bed. If they're not, keep practicing until they are.

Take every day, every meal, one step at a time. You don't have to lose fifty pounds overnight. Just have a nice breakfast. Eat your soup for lunch. Keep your fitness date and take a walk after a delicious dinner.

If it's not fun, don't do it. Hateful things are not on the Path. If a person, a practice, or a behavior brings you happiness, joy, serenity, and calm, keep it in your life. If something or someone bums you out, avoid it.

Keep calm and C.H.A.N.G.E. on! My objective has never been to create a "diet you can live with forever." (A forever diet? Shoot me now.) My goal is to help women restore radiant health, balance, energy, flexibility, and well-being in a self-sustaining way. The healthier you are, the better you feel, the happier you are, the more you want to stay that way. Everything you've learned in the last eight weeks is yours to keep. Your body was born to move, and now you'll reap the benefits of homeostasis for as long as you keep up the good work. Congrats on everything you've done, no matter how small, to gain knowledge, wisdom, and health. It's been my honor and privilege to be your guide. But now I have to wave you ahead and ask you to take the lead. Your Path is your own. Hike your own hike, in good health, warm sunshine, and comfortable shoes.

PART FOUR

Start Souping

22.

The Recipes

My soups are as nutritious as they are delicious. But you can't get this many nutrients into a stockpot without chopping a lot of vegetables, so sharpen your knives, women. For some of my patients, making soup is a little bit of a challenge at first. The women who struggle most are usually inexperienced cooks who are intimidated by the amount of prep work that goes into making soup from scratch. But there is no success in life or in soup without experience. When it comes to soup, you just have to learn to measure accurately, chop roughly, and simmer for an extended time. And then, you're golden.

By Week Three, everyone on the Path becomes a "souper star." If you feel at all intimidated by the number of ingredients or by one you might not have heard of yet, do a quick round of pranayama breathing and relax. You have nothing to fear from a vegetable. Every new ingredient you work with will soon become an old friend.

Split Pea Soup

Makes 12 servings

1 tablespoon coconut oil
2 medium raw onions, diced
Sea salt
3 cups diced raw celery stalks
3 cups diced raw carrots
10 cloves raw garlic, minced, or 2 tablespoons jarred minced garlic
3 tablespoons finely minced fresh sage or 1 tablespoon ground sage
4 teaspoons finely minced fresh thyme or 1⅓ teaspoons dried thyme
3 cups diced parsnips
½ head cauliflower, finely diced
2 cups diced broccoli rabe
1 cup dried mung beans, soaked overnight
1½ cups dried split peas, soaked overnight
2 cups uncooked quinoa
1 cup whole flax seeds
Freshly ground black pepper

INSTRUCTIONS

In a large stockpot over medium heat, place the coconut oil. When the oil has liquefied, add the onions and 1 teaspoon of salt. Stir until the onions are translucent, 3 to 4 minutes.

Add the celery, stirring until slightly softened, 3 to 4 minutes. Then add the carrots, stirring until slightly softened, 3 to 5 minutes.

Stir in the garlic, sage, and thyme. Add the parsnips and stir until slightly softened, 3 to 5 minutes. Then add the cauliflower, stirring again until slightly softened, 3 to 5 minutes. Add the broccoli rabe and stir until slightly softened, about 3 minutes.

Add 10 of cups of water and bring to simmer.

Add the mung beans and simmer until softened, about 10 minutes. Then add the split peas and simmer until softened, about 5 minutes.

Add 3 cups of water, or fill to an inch below the rim of the pot, and return to a simmer.

Add the quinoa, stirring until cooked, about 7 minutes. The quinoa will look like it has a curlicue coming out of it and should be soft to the bite.

Add the flax seeds.

Salt and pepper can be added to taste in the individual servings.

Chattanooga Chili

Makes 12 servings

1 tablespoon coconut oil
2 medium raw yellow onions, diced
Salt
2 cups diced celery stalks
3 cups diced raw carrots
12 cloves raw garlic, minced, or 3 tablespoons jarred minced garlic
1 or 2 raw jalapeño peppers, seeded and finely diced
2 cups okra, cut into ½-inch slices
2 medium raw green bell peppers, diced
2 cups chopped raw spinach
1 cup finely chopped fresh cilantro
6 cups canned tomatoes or 8 cups diced fresh tomatoes
3 tablespoons chili powder
3 teaspoons ground turmeric
3 tablespoons ground cumin
½ to 1 teaspoon cayenne pepper
2 tablespoons organic olive oil
1 package frozen organic corn
2 medium raw red bell peppers, diced
2½ cups cooked black-eyed peas
3¾ cups cooked black beans
1¾ cups cooked kidney beans
2½ cups cooked white beans
2½ tablespoons flax seeds
6 tablespoons hemp seeds
Freshly ground black pepper

INSTRUCTIONS

In a large stockpot over medium heat, place the coconut oil. When the oil has liquefied, add the onions and 1 teaspoon of salt and stir until the onions are translucent, 3 to 5 minutes.

Add the celery and stir until slightly softened, 3 to 4 minutes. Then add the carrots and stir until softened, 3 to 5 minutes.

Stir in the garlic and 1 or 2 (depending on how hot you like it) jalapeños. Add the okra and green bell peppers and continue to cook, stirring until softened, 3 to 4 minutes.

Add the spinach and cilantro and stir until wilted, 2 to 3 minutes. Add the tomatoes and stir. Then add the chili powder, turmeric, and cumin. Stir well. Add the cayenne to taste (½ teaspoon for mild to 1 teaspoon or more for spicy).

Add 10 cups of water, or fill to approximately 2 inches below the rim of the pot, and the olive oil; stir thoroughly and simmer until softened, about 15 minutes.

Add the corn and red bell peppers and simmer for 5 minutes.

Add the black-eyed peas and all the beans, the flax seeds, and the hemp seeds. Cook until heated through. Season with salt and pepper to taste.

Green Chili Hominy Stew

Makes 12 servings

8 large mild green peppers, such as Anaheim chile peppers, or 8 cans
    mild roasted green peppers (see roasting instructions below if using
    fresh peppers)
2 tablespoons coconut oil
2 medium raw onions, diced
Salt
2 cups diced celery stalks
3 cups diced medium carrots
10 cloves raw garlic, minced
Freshly ground black pepper
3 cups chopped raw okra
½ cup finely chopped fresh cilantro
12 cups chopped raw spinach
3 cups diced fresh or canned (with juice) tomatillos
2 cups raw mung beans
3 teaspoons ground cumin
2 large red bell peppers, chopped
1 tablespoon olive oil
4 tablespoons flax seeds
2 (28-ounce) cans white hominy (Juanita's brand is non-GMO)
For a "flexitarian" version you can substitute up to 3 cups shredded
    poached organic chicken breast for 1 can of white hominy

INSTRUCTIONS

Roast the whole green peppers by placing them on a baking sheet
in the oven under the broiler. Flip them with kitchen tongs when
one side becomes just blackened and repeat until all sides are equally
roasted. Remove the peppers from the oven and place them in a brown

paper bag. After approximately 5 minutes, when cool enough to handle, the skins and stems can be easily removed. For less spicy peppers, remove the seeds as well. Dice and set aside.

In a stockpot over medium heat, place the coconut oil. When the oil has liquefied, add the onions and a pinch of salt. Stir occasionally until the onions are soft and translucent, 3 to 4 minutes.

Add the celery and stir until softened, about 3 minutes. Then add the carrots and stir until softened, 3 to 5 minutes.

Add the garlic and stir. Add 3 to 4 grinds (about 1 teaspoon) of black pepper to the mixture. Then add the okra and stir occasionally until softened, about 3 minutes.

Add the cilantro and stir. Then add the spinach and stir occasionally until wilted, about 1 minute. Add the tomatillos and crush them into smaller pieces with a wooden spoon. Stir until incorporated.

Add 6 cups of water and bring to a simmer.

Stir in the mung beans and simmer until the beans are soft, about 10 minutes. Add the cumin and stir.

Add an additional 4 cups of water, or fill to about 2 inches below the rim of the pot, and bring to a simmer.

Add the red peppers, olive oil, and flax seeds and simmer for 5 minutes. Stir in the hominy and roasted chiles, and cook for 5 to 7 minutes until warmed throughout. Remove 3 cups of soup from the pot. Then, in a standard blender or with an immersion blender, pulse until lightly blended but not completely pureed, and return to the stockpot still on the stove. Add in the chicken, if using. Stir and bring to a simmer.

Add salt and pepper to taste to individual servings.

Enchilada Soup

Makes 12 servings

1 tablespoon coconut oil

2 cups diced raw onions

Salt

2 cups diced celery

12 garlic cloves, minced, or 2 tablespoons jarred minced garlic

2 cups diced carrots

1 head cauliflower, diced

1½ cups diced green bell peppers

3 cups chopped spinach

1 cup finely chopped cilantro

7 cups canned chopped tomatoes (with juice) or 3 pounds fresh
    tomatoes, diced

1 tablespoon olive oil

2 cups diced sweet potatoes

2 cups diced beets

1 cup dry adzuki beans, soaked overnight

3 cups hominy (Juanita's brand is non-GMO)

3 cups (approximately 1 pound) shredded poached organic chicken
    breast

2 teaspoons harissa seasoning or to taste

3 cups cooked black beans

1½ cups diced red bell peppers

¼ cup hemp seeds

¾ cup flax seeds

INSTRUCTIONS

In a stockpot over medium heat, place the coconut oil. When the oil
has liquefied, add the onions, sprinkle with 1 teaspoon salt, and stir
until the onions are translucent, 2 to 3 minutes.

Add the celery and stir occasionally until softened, 2 to 3 minutes. Then add the garlic and stir for 1 minute. Add the carrots, stirring occasionally, and cook for 3 to 5 minutes until softened. Then add the cauliflower and stir about 3 minutes, until softened.

Add the green peppers and stir, about 3 minutes. Then add the spinach and stir until wilted, about 1 minute. Add the cilantro and stir, about 1 minute. Then add the chopped tomatoes with the juice and stir until incorporated.

Add 6 cups of water, or fill to approximately 2 inches below the rim of the pot. Then add the olive oil, stir thoroughly, and bring the soup to a simmer.

Stir in the sweet potatoes, beets, and adzuki beans. Let simmer until the adzuki beans are soft, 10 to 15 minutes.

Add the hominy, chicken, and harissa seasoning and stir thoroughly. Then add the black beans, red peppers, hemp seeds, and flax seeds. Simmer, stirring occasionally, for another 5 to 7 minutes.

Add salt and pepper to taste to individual servings.

French Onion Soup

Makes 12 servings

2 cooked spaghetti squash

1 tablespoon coconut oil

12 garlic cloves, minced, or 2 tablespoons jarred minced garlic

6 onions, thinly sliced

Salt

3 tablespoons balsamic vinegar

5 cups carrots, cut into thin strips with a potato peeler

4 stalks celery, cut into thin strips with a potato peeler or food
    processor

2 tablespoons fresh thyme

2 cups parsnips, roughly chopped into 1-inch pieces

2 cups sweet potatoes (purple ones are fun), roughly chopped into
    1-inch pieces

2 cups green zucchini, skin on, chopped into ½-inch pieces

2 cups yellow zucchini, skin on, chopped into ½-inch pieces

1 tablespoon olive oil

4 one-quart cartons organic beef or vegetable broth

1½ cups quinoa

½ cup hemp seeds

¼ cup hemp powder

4 tablespoons nutritional yeast

1 cup grated Gruyere cheese

1 cup grated Parmigiano-Reggiano cheese

Freshly ground black pepper

*FOR A VEGAN VERSION, OMIT THE CHEESE AND
REPLACE WITH THE SAUCE BELOW:*

4 cups cooked cauliflower

4 cups soup broth

1 cup nutritional yeast

1 tablespoon salt
½ teaspoon paprika
¼ teaspoon turmeric
½ tablespoon Dijon mustard

In a blender, blend all ingredients on high until smooth.

INSTRUCTIONS

Preheat the oven to 400° F. To cook the spaghetti squash, do not peel the squash. Cut them in half lengthwise and remove the seeds from the center. Place cut-sides down in a medium baking dish with 1 inch of water. Bake in the oven for approximately 40 minutes, until you can just pierce the skin of the squash with a fork. Let rest 15 minutes. Be careful not to overcook the squash. Remove the squash from the oven and let cool. Use a fork to scrape the insides from the squash, and set aside.

In a stockpot over medium heat, place the coconut oil and heat until liquefied. Add the garlic and sauté until aromatic. Then add the onions and sprinkle with 1 teaspoon salt. Cook for 3 minutes until slightly softened.

Add the balsamic vinegar and stir until slightly caramelized, 5 to 7 minutes. Add the carrots and celery and stir until slightly softened, 2 to 3 minutes. Stir in the thyme. Add the parsnips and stir until slightly softened.

Add the sweet potatoes and stir until slightly softened, 2 to 3 minutes. Then add all the zucchini and stir until slightly softened, 2 to 3 minutes. Add the olive oil and stir to thoroughly incorporate.

Add the broth and bring to a simmer. Then add the quinoa and cook until the quinoa is cooked, 10 to 15 minutes. Add the hemp seeds, hemp powder, and yeast. Stir to incorporate.

Stir in the cheeses or vegan cheese sauce (see variation above) and cook until fully incorporated, about 5 minutes.

Add salt and pepper to taste.

Corn Chowder Two Ways

Makes 12 servings

1 tablespoon coconut oil
2 cups diced yellow onions
2 cups diced carrots
2 cups diced celery
2 cups diced parsnips
12 cloves of garlic, minced
2 cups diced potatoes
2 cups quinoa
4 cups spinach
3½ cups organic corn (may use frozen)
Cauliflower puree (see below)
2 cups hemp seeds
Salt and freshly ground black pepper

FOR CAULIFLOWER PUREE:
1 head steamed cauliflower florets
¾ cup nutritional yeast
1 cup milk or unsweetened milk alternative
1 cup water
One ½-inch slice lemon with peel, no seeds

FOR HERBED CORN CHOWDER:
2 tablespoons fresh thyme

FOR SOUTHWESTERN CORN CHOWDER:
2 cups finely chopped cilantro
2 cups diced red bell peppers
2 cups (about 6 jars) roasted green chiles
2 tablespoons Tabasco sauce or to taste

INSTRUCTIONS

In a stockpot over medium heat, place the coconut oil and heat until liquefied. Add the onions and sauté until the onions are just translucent.

Add the carrots and stir until slightly softened, 3 to 4 minutes. Then add the celery and stir until slightly softened, 3 to 4 minutes. Add the parsnips and stir until slightly softened, 3 to 4 minutes. Then add the garlic and stir to incorporate.

Add 11 cups of water and stir thoroughly. Bring to a simmer.

Add the potatoes and cook until slightly softened, about 10 minutes. Then add the quinoa and cook for another 10 minutes. Add the spinach, corn, and cauliflower puree and stir to incorporate thoroughly.

To make the cauliflower puree: In a blender, blend together all the ingredients.

For Herbed Corn Chowder: Add thyme and hemp seeds, stirring thoroughly, until heated through. Add salt and pepper to taste.

For Southwestern Corn Chowder: Add the cilantro and hemp seeds and stir to incorporate. Then add the red peppers and the green chiles and stir thoroughly until heated through. Add the Tabasco and salt and pepper to taste.

Sriracha Brussels Sprout Soup

Makes 12 servings

7½ cups quartered Brussels sprouts
2 tablespoons coconut oil
3 tablespoons minced garlic
2 cups diced celery
2 cups diced carrots
1 cup chopped cilantro
6 cups chopped spinach
12 cups low-sodium organic vegetable or chicken broth
Two 7-ounce packages mung bean/edamame pasta (available at
    Amazon Prime or Whole Foods in the Asian foods section)
1 tablespoon olive oil
9 tablespoons honey
1 to 3 tablespoons Sriracha
3 large limes
Salt
For a "flexitarian" version, you can add as much as 3 cups poached
    shredded organic chicken breast meat, if desired.

INSTRUCTIONS

Toss the Brussels sprouts with 1 tablespoon liquefied coconut oil and
roast on medium in the oven on a baking sheet under the broiler for 5
to 10 minutes, or until browned all over. They may need to be stirred
midway. Set aside.

Heat the remaining tablespoon of coconut oil in a soup pot until
liquefied, then add the garlic. Once the garlic is aromatic, stir in the
celery and sauté until slightly softened, about 3 minutes.

Add the carrots and cook until slightly softened, 3 to 5 minutes. Stir in the cilantro to incorporate. Add the chopped spinach and stir until slightly wilted, 2 to 3 minutes.

Add the broth to the pot and bring to a simmer. Add the mung bean pasta and olive oil and simmer until the pasta is al dente, 5 to 7 minutes.

While the pasta is cooking, in a small bowl, stir together the honey, Sriracha, and the juice of one lime. Once the pasta is cooked, add the honey mixture and stir well, about 3 minutes.

Add the reserved Brussels sprouts and chicken, if using, and stir to incorporate.

Add salt and more Sriracha to taste, if desired. Serve with lime wedges.

Indian Dal Soup

Makes 12 servings

1 tablespoon coconut oil
2 large onions, diced
1 cup diced celery
2 cups diced carrots
1 head cauliflower, chopped into bite-size pieces
3 cups quartered Brussels sprouts
2 cups diced zucchini, skin on
8 cups chopped spinach
2 quarts vegetable broth
4 cups water
2 cups diced sweet potatoes
2 teaspoons curry powder
2 tablespoons garam masala seasoning powder
4 tablespoons ginger (I used the minced jar kind, but you can use fresh;
    you may need to adjust the recipe to taste, though)
2 cups dried lentils, soaked overnight
4 cups cooked garbanzo beans
Salt and freshly ground black pepper

INSTRUCTIONS

In a stockpot over medium heat, place the coconut oil and heat until liquefied. Add the onions and sauté until the onions are translucent, 2 to 3 minutes.

Add the celery and stir until softened, 2 to 3 minutes. Then add the carrots and stir until softened, 2 to 3 minutes. Add the cauliflower and stir until softened, 3 to 5 minutes. Then add the Brussels sprouts and stir until softened, 2 to 3 minutes. Add the zucchini and stir until softened, 2 to 3 minutes. Then add the spinach and stir until wilted, 1 to 2 minutes.

Add the broth and water and bring to a simmer. Add the sweet potatoes, curry powder, garam masala, and ginger and stir well to incorporate. Once the sweet potatoes have softened, in 10 to 15 minutes, add the lentils and cook until the lentils are soft. Add the garbanzo beans and stir.

Add salt and pepper to taste.

Broccoli Cheddar Soup Two Ways

Makes 12 servings

1 tablespoon coconut oil
2 medium onions, diced
Salt
3 cups diced celery
12 cloves garlic, minced, or 3 tablespoons jarred minced garlic
3 cups diced carrots
1 tablespoon finely chopped fresh thyme, no stems
2 teaspoons Dijon mustard
1 tablespoon olive oil
6 cups chopped broccoli florets, cut into bite-size pieces
3 cups chopped cauliflower, cut into bite-size pieces
6 cups thinly chopped kale
2 cups cubed potatoes, cut into bite-size pieces
1 teaspoon ground nutmeg
12 teaspoons whole flax seeds
1 cup uncooked quinoa
1½ cups uncooked lentils, soaked overnight
2 cups shredded cheddar cheese
1 cup shredded Parmesan cheese
Freshly ground black pepper

NON-DAIRY VERSION, OMIT THE CHEESE AND SUBSTITUTE THE FOLLOWING INGREDIENTS:
1½ cups nutritional yeast
1 tablespoon freshly squeezed lemon juice
1 cup raw unsalted cashew nuts

INSTRUCTIONS

In a stockpot over medium heat, place the coconut oil and heat until just liquefied. Add the onions, sprinkle with 1 teaspoon of salt, and stir occasionally until the onions are translucent, 2 to 3 minutes.

Add the celery and stir occasionally until softened, 2 to 3 minutes. Then add the garlic and stir until aromatic, about 1 minute. Add the carrots, stirring occasionally, about 5 minutes, until the carrots soften. Then add the thyme and Dijon mustard and stir to incorporate.

Add 4 cups of water and the olive oil and stir to incorporate. Bring to a simmer and then add the broccoli and cauliflower, stirring occasionally for 5 minutes until the broccoli and cauliflower have softened slightly. Add the kale and stir until wilted, about 3 minutes.

Add 10 cups of water, or fill to about 2 inches below the rim of the pot, and return to a simmer while stirring occasionally.

Add the potatoes and simmer, stirring intermittently, until just softened, about 10 minutes. Add the nutmeg and flax seeds and stir to incorporate.

Add the quinoa and lentils and simmer until cooked, 10 to 15 minutes.

Once cooked, remove 4 cups of the soup and set aside until slightly cooled, 2 cups at a time, then place in a blender and blend until just smooth. Do not overblend, or the soup will become too thin. Add half the cheddar cheese and half the Parmesan to the blender and pulse blend on high until the cheeses are incorporated. Repeat with the other 2 cups. (All 4 cups can be done at once with an immersion blender by adding the cheeses to the reserved soup and blending until the cheeses are incorporated.) Return the blended portions to the pot and stir for 5 to 7 minutes until the cheeses are melted and the soup is heated through. Add salt and pepper to taste.

For the non-dairy version: Remove only 1 cup of the soup and place in the blender, adding the nutritional yeast, lemon juice, and cashews. Blend on high until smooth. Return the blended portion to the pot and stir to fully incorporate. Add salt and pepper to taste.

Rosemary Mushroom Soup

Makes 12 servings

2 cups uncooked freekeh or spelt (or, for a gluten-free version,
    use 1 cup buckwheat and 1 cup quinoa)
1 tablespoon coconut oil
2 medium onions, diced
Salt
3 cups diced celery
3 cups diced carrots
12 cloves garlic
2 tablespoons fresh thyme or 2 teaspoons dried thyme
4 tablespoons fresh rosemary, very finely minced, plus one fresh sprig
2 cups diced yams
14 cups diced mushrooms
1 large head cauliflower, finely chopped
6 cups finely chopped kale
1 tablespoon olive oil
1 cup uncooked amaranth
3½ cups cooked no-salt-added artichoke hearts in water, divided
3 cups cooked white beans, divided
4 tablespoons chia seeds
Salt and freshly ground black pepper

INSTRUCTIONS

If using freekeh or spelt, fill a separate pot with 7 cups of water and
bring to a boil. Add the freekeh or spelt and cook on low for 1 hour or
until it is the consistency of cooked rice. You may need to add a little
water during the cooking process, as the grain can absorb a lot.

While waiting for the freekeh or spelt to cook, in a stockpot over medium heat, place the coconut oil and heat until liquefied. Add the onions and stir until translucent, 3 to 5 minutes.

Add the celery and stir occasionally until slightly softened, about 3 minutes. Then add the carrots and stir until softened, about 5 minutes. Add the garlic, thyme, and sprig of rosemary and stir to combine.

Add the yams and stir until softened, 3 to 5 minutes. Then add the mushrooms and stir until softened, about 5 minutes. Add the cauliflower and stir until softened, 3 to 5 minutes. Then add the kale and stir until wilted, 1 to 2 minutes. Remove the rosemary sprig and set aside.

Add 10 cups of water and the olive oil and stir to incorporate. Bring to a simmer.

Add the 4 tablespoons of fresh rosemary and stir to combine. Then add the cooked freekeh or spelt (for a gluten-free version, add the uncooked buckwheat and uncooked quinoa) and simmer until it has the consistency of cooked rice. Add the amaranth. Stir well and return to a simmer.

Put half the artichoke hearts, beans, and chia seeds in a blender and pulse blend on high for 10 short pulses or until just blended together. Do not overblend. Add the mixture to the stockpot and stir to incorporate. Repeat with the other half.

Add salt and pepper to taste.

Thai Coconut Soup

Makes 12 servings

1 tablespoon coconut oil
2 medium onions, diced
Salt
3 cups diced celery
3 cups diced carrots
2 cups okra, cut crosswise into ½ inch slices
1 tablespoon olive oil
4 cups chopped broccoli florets or broccoli rabe, cut into bite-size pieces
12 cloves garlic, minced, or 6 teaspoons jarred minced garlic
1 or 2 jalapeño peppers, seeded and minced
8 teaspoons fresh grated ginger root or minced from a jar
1 tablespoon fresh lemon zest
8 cups chopped kale
1 cup chopped fresh cilantro
16 shiitake (or comparable) mushrooms, chopped
5 tablespoons freshly squeezed lime juice (2½ limes)
4 tablespoons fish sauce
3 tablespoons tahini
1 cup uncooked wild rice
2½ cups uncooked mung beans, soaked overnight
1½ cups unsweetened coconut milk
1 cup uncooked amaranth grain
1 medium red bell pepper, sliced
⅓ cup sesame seeds
Freshly ground black pepper

INSTRUCTIONS

In a stockpot over medium heat, place the coconut oil and heat until liquefied. Add the onions and a pinch of salt and stir until the onions are translucent, about 3 minutes.

Add the celery and stir until softened, about 3 minutes. Then add the carrots and stir until softened, about 5 minutes. Add the okra and stir until softened, about 3 minutes.

Add 2 cups of hot water and the olive oil and stir to combine. Add the broccoli and stir until slightly softened, about 3 minutes. Then add the garlic, jalapeños (1 for mild and 2 for spicy), ginger root, and lemon zest and stir to incorporate.

Add the kale and stir until wilted, about 1 minute. Then add the cilantro and stir until wilted, about 1 minute. Add the mushrooms and stir until softened, 3 to 5 minutes. Stir in the lime juice and fish sauce. Add the tahini and continue stirring.

Add 12 cups of water, or fill to approximately 3 inches below the rim of the pot, and bring to a simmer. Add the rice and mung beans and simmer for about 30 minutes. Add the coconut milk and water, if needed, to approximately 1 inch below the rim of the pot and return to a simmer. Add the amaranth and simmer until cooked, about 10 minutes. Then add the red pepper and simmer for another 5 minutes. Add the sesame seeds and salt and pepper to taste.

Shrimp Bisque

Makes 12 servings

1 tablespoon coconut oil
2 medium onions, chopped
Salt
3 cups chopped celery
3 cups chopped carrots
12 cloves garlic, minced, or 6 teaspoons jarred minced garlic
1 large head cauliflower, diced
4 cups chopped spinach
1 fennel bulb, diced
¾ cup fish sauce
1½ teaspoons paprika
1 teaspoon turmeric
1 cup whole flax seeds
1 cup uncooked lentils
3 cups farro or buckwheat (if gluten-free)
1 cup uncooked quinoa
36 medium wild shrimp (scallops may be substituted), cooked and diced
½ cup finely chopped fresh dill or more to taste
3½ cups canned diced tomatoes (with juice) or 4 cups diced fresh ripe
    tomatoes
Freshly ground black pepper

INSTRUCTIONS

In a large stockpot over medium heat, place the coconut oil and heat until slightly liquefied. Add the onions and a pinch of salt and stir until the onions are translucent.

Add the celery and stir until softened, about 3 minutes. Then add the carrots and stir until softened, 3 to 5 minutes. Add the garlic, cauliflower, spinach, and fennel and stir until softened. Then add the fish sauce and stir to combine, 5 to 7 minutes, until softened. Add 12 cups of water, or fill to approximately 2 inches below the rim of the pot, and stir. Add the paprika, turmeric, and flax seeds. Stir and bring to a simmer.

Add the lentils and stir occasionally until al dente. (The lentils will absorb water, so add more, as needed, to reach 1 inch below the rim of the pot.) Return to a simmer.

Add the farro or buckwheat and stir occasionally until al dente, about 15 minutes. Add the quinoa and more water to again fill the pot to 1 inch from the rim. Stir occasionally and simmer until the lentils and farro are cooked, about 20 minutes.

Remove 4 cups of the soup from the pot, 2 cups at a time. Let cool for 2 to 3 minutes, then blend in a blender for 15 seconds or use an immersion blender to blend all 4 cups at once. Return the blended mixture to the pot. If using a blender, repeat with the other 2 cups. Add the fresh dill and stir.

In the meantime, steam the shrimp or scallops until just done. If you don't have a steamer basket, you can use a metal colander. Place the whole shrimp in their shells into the colander and place the colander over a pot of boiling water. Choose a pot big enough for the colander to nestle about halfway into the pot. The water level in the pot should be slightly below the bottom of the colander. Cover the colander with the pot lid for 5 to 6 minutes, stirring once after 2 minutes. Shrimp are done when they just turn opaque and are firm to the touch. Remove them from the colander, and when cool enough to handle, peel them, then mince. Add the cooked shrimp to the soup pot and stir to incorporate.

Add salt and pepper to taste.

Roasted Squash and Apple Soup

Makes 12 servings

12 cups cubed raw butternut squash (cut into 1-inch cubes)
3 cups unpeeled cubed firm sweet apples like Mcintosh or Fuji
    (cut into 1-inch cubes)
2 cups quartered Brussels sprouts
2 tablespoons coconut oil at room temperature (liquid)
Salt
2 teaspoons cumin
2 medium onions, 1 diced, 1 quartered
3 cups diced celery
3 cups diced carrots
12 cloves raw garlic, minced, or 6 teaspoons jarred minced garlic
    (divided)
1 tablespoon minced fresh thyme or 3 teaspoons dried thyme
2 tablespoons minced fresh sage or 6 teaspoons dried sage
1 cup finely chopped kale
2½ cups uncooked quinoa
1 cup whole flax seeds
4 tablespoons chia seeds
Freshly ground black pepper
1 tablespoon of shelled pumpkin seeds, for garnish

INSTRUCTIONS

Toss the squash, apples, and Brussels sprouts together with 1 table-spoon of the coconut oil, a pinch of salt, and half the garlic and place on a large rimmed baking sheet in the oven on the lowest shelf. Add water to about ¼ inch deep to create a moist roasting environment. Loosely cover with tinfoil and place on the middle rack of the oven under the broiler on high. Roast squash and sprouts until softened, but not browned, approximately 7 to 10 minutes. The squash should be easy to pierce with a fork. In a blender, place 1 cup of water, the cumin, and 1 cup of the roasted squash and apple mixture and puree. Repeat with the remaining mixture. Set aside.

In a stockpot over medium heat, heat the remaining tablespoon of the coconut oil. When the oil is liquified, add the diced onions, the garlic, and a pinch of salt. Stir until the vegetables are translucent, about 3 minutes.

Add the celery and stir until softened, about 3 minutes. Then add the carrots and stir until softened, 5 to 7 minutes. Add the thyme and sage and stir. Then add the kale and stir until wilted, 1 to 2 minutes.

Add 12 cups of water to the pot and bring to a simmer. Add the quinoa and flax seeds and simmer until the quinoa is tender, 10 to 15 minutes. Add the chia seeds.

Remove the pot from the heat, add the reserved squash and apple puree, and stir. Add salt and pepper to taste and garnish with the pumpkin seeds.

Anna's Ratatouille Soup

Anna has been a patient of mine for fifteen years. She is an amazing woman and came up with this delicious soup version of one of her favorite French meals. Bon appétit!

Makes 6 servings

1 diced green zucchini
1 diced yellow zucchini
1 diced medium unpeeled eggplant (about the size of a grapefruit)
1 diced red bell pepper
1 diced yellow bell pepper
1 tablespoon coconut oil (leave at room temperature until liquefied)
Salt and freshly ground black pepper
4 cloves garlic, minced
2 diced onions
3 cups finely chopped Swiss chard, tough stems removed
1 32-ounce carton low-sodium organic vegetable or chicken broth
3 cups canned tomatoes or 4 cups fresh tomatoes
1 cup finely chopped fresh basil
1 tablespoon fresh oregano or 1 teaspoon dried oregano
1 tablespoon fresh Italian parsley or 1 teaspoon dried parsley
1 cup farro
1 cup quinoa
2 tablespoons hemp seeds

INSTRUCTIONS

Dice all the vegetables except the Swiss chard, toss them with the coconut oil and garlic, and season with salt and pepper. Place the vegetables on a baking sheet in the oven under the broiler. Roast until the vegetables begin to brown.

In a stockpot over medium heat, place the coconut oil and heat until liquefied. Add the garlic and onions and stir until translucent, 3 to 5 minutes. Add the roasted vegetables, stirring until soft, 5 to 7 minutes. Add the Swiss chard and stir until wilted, about 3 minutes. Add the vegetable broth, 2 additional cups of water, the tomatoes, and the herbs and bring to simmer. Add the farro and cook for 20 minutes, until al dente. Add the quinoa and cook for 15 minutes. Stir in the hemp seeds until incorporated.

Tracy's Chinese Takeout Soup

Before Tracy got on the Well Path, Chinese takeout was a quick go-to when she was superhungry after working long hours without lunch or after going to the gym on an empty stomach. In her recipe, she re-created the flavor she loves that is full of nutritional bang!

Makes 10 servings

2 tablespoons coconut oil
12 cloves raw garlic, minced
3 cups chopped celery
1 pound wild shrimp, steamed and minced
4 cups chopped broccoli
2½ cups chopped bok choy
2½ cups shredded carrots
2 tablespoons honey
4 tablespoons chopped cilantro
4 tablespoons minced fresh or jarred ginger
1 cup finely chopped scallions
1½ cups quinoa
6 tablespoons flax seeds
6 tablespoons sesame seeds
Salt and freshly ground black pepper

INSTRUCTIONS

In a stockpot over low heat, heat the coconut oil, then add the garlic and stir until slightly browned.

Add the celery and stir, 3 to 5 minutes.

Meanwhile, steam the shrimp until just done. If you don't have a steamer basket, you can use a metal colander. Place the whole shrimp in their shells into the colander and place the colander over a pot of boiling water. Choose a pot big enough for the colander to nestle about halfway into the pot. The water level in the pot should be just below the bottom of the colander. Cover the colander with the pot lid for 5 to 6 minutes, stirring once after 2 minutes. Shrimp are done when they just turn opaque. Remove them from the colander, let cool until easy to handle, peel them, and then mince. Set aside.

While the shrimp is cooking, add 2 cups of water to the pot and bring to a simmer. Add the broccoli and bok choy and cook for 5 to 7 minutes, until softened. Then stir in the carrots.

Add 6 cups of water and the honey and bring to a simmer. Add the shrimp, cilantro, and ginger and stir to combine.

Add 4 more cups of water to the pot. Add the scallions and stir until wilted. Then add the quinoa, flax seeds, and sesame seeds and return to a simmer for 15 minutes.

Add salt and pepper to taste.

Gina's Buffalo Chicken Soup

When I first met Gina, she had no idea how to cook anything that wasn't in a box. That Gina is long gone! One of her favorite foods when eating out is Buffalo chicken wings, so she used her creative, "go get 'em" spirit to make a nutritious soup that satisfies.

Makes 6 servings

1 large head cauliflower, cut into florets
Tabasco or Sriracha sauce to taste
2 tablespoons olive oil
1 medium onion, diced
2 tablespoons minced garlic
5 stalks celery, diced
1 pound carrots, diced
3 cups chopped spinach
1 cup quinoa
½ pound poached chicken, shredded
6 tablespoons hemp seeds for garnish (1 tablespoon per serving)

RANCH SEASONING
2 tablespoons dried parsley
2 teaspoons dried dill
1 teaspoon garlic powder
1 teaspoon onion powder
½ teaspoon black pepper
½ teaspoon dried chives
Pinch of salt
1 cup Greek yogurt

INSTRUCTIONS

Steam the cauliflower by placing the florets in a steamer basket or metal colander in or over a boiling pot of water. Cover the pot or colander with a lid. Steam for 5 to 7 minutes until tender. In a blender, place 1 cup of the water from the pot, the cauliflower, and the Tabasco sauce to taste and blend on medium into a puree. Or place the cauliflower, Tabasco, and water into a bowl and use an immersion blender to puree to a smooth or almost smooth consistency.

To make the ranch seasoning, add the dried parsley through Greek yogurt to the cauliflower puree and blend on medium until smooth.

In a stockpot, over medium heat, place the oil and the onion, garlic, celery, and carrots. Stir until the vegetables are soft, 5 to 7 minutes. Then add the spinach and stir for 2 to 3 minutes, until wilted.

Add 7 cups of water to the stockpot. Then add the quinoa and bring to a simmer for 20 minutes. Once the quinoa is cooked, add the chicken. Stir in the cauliflower mixture and heat all the way through on medium for 5 to 7 minutes. Add salt and pepper to taste.

Garnish with hemp seeds.

Acknowledgments

It is with immeasurable gratitude that I sit here typing the acknowledgments for this book. Being the trusted ear for thousands of women through the decades of their life is indeed the greatest privilege. So first and foremost, I must acknowledge the women in my practice who put their trust in me every day and who have given their support and care when I needed them in return.

A very special acknowledgment must go to the twenty-three women who graciously and enthusiastically allowed me to document their journey on the Well Path for this book. Together we cooked soup on Sundays, hiked in knee-deep snow, and ran through Central Park in freezing temperatures. We bounced, jazzed, Zumba'd, climbed, and yoga'd for sixty days during one of the coldest winters on record. But, most of all, we encouraged one another unconditionally toward our common goal . . . life C.H.A.N.G.E. And we *did* change. It was one of the most gratifying sixty-day periods of my life, and their experiences helped shape this book. If you were able to find transformation within the pages of this book, it is a direct reflection of their journey.

Maisy, Diane, Gina, Anna, Sulekha, Catherine, Mary, Wren, Tracy, Alaké, Alona, Denise, Emily, Royda, Joanne, Carolyn, Lana, Renee, Heather, Erika, Filomena, Melanie, and Yvonne, *you* are my SouperStars.

My journey with these women would not have been possible without several people at home, at work, and at the fitness venues that supported this project.

First and foremost, thank you to Krisztina Szep and Jessica Costa for always responding enthusiastically to my sometimes last-minute panicked calls for help at home when I couldn't be at two (or three) places at once. I hope you know how much I appreciate your being so loyal and loving to my family. Thanks go to Laura D'amico, who was immensely helpful with the logistics of this program, including getting up at the crack of dawn for the fifteen-hour Soup Sundays and responding valiantly every time I said, "Oops, I forgot something." Thank you to Lalo Fuentes of Lalo Fitness for his expert advice and for graciously lending his time for the instructional videos we produced for the book's website. Thank you to Lori Sanchez Abeles, spinning instructor extraordinaire at Soul Cycle, who enthusiastically gifted her time to take my ladies on a special ride to celebrate the success of their Well Path journey. It was a great moment of esteem for these women, and to have Lori at the helm was particularly meaningful for me, given my own weight-loss journey with her. And thank you to Andrea Borrero and Jon Witt of Pure Yoga—Andrea for arranging classes for the ladies, and Jon for his expert and kind support in teaching the beginners.

Special gratitude goes to Susan Woods of Woods & Co. for offering me so many opportunities to reach out to the public with my message.

With gratitude to Claire Mercury for her support and enthusiasm in promoting this book.

My own journey to this book has been a series of uphill climbs and forks in the road. My destination might have been quite different if I hadn't had the good fortune to have met some very special people on my path. Thank you to my high school volleyball coach, Mike Lynn, for the tough love and advice at a critical point in my life that have resonated with me over the years in times of great physical or mental challenge. I still visualize that "brick wall" when I need to dig deep and power through. Your wise words nudged me toward the path of perseverance.

Thank you to my mentor Janet Hopkins, for her unwavering support during my residency at Swedish Medical Center. When others were telling me my entrepreneurial endeavors were a sure waste of my medical training, she told me to listen to myself and trust my instincts to practice medicine outside of the box. She also imparted this powerful mantra: "There are many ways to heal people." To me, this is the essence of being a doctor. In the absence of concrete answers, this mantra has guided me to just holding a hand or listening as a powerful way of healing.

Thank you to Shivaun Mahoney, who for the past twelve years has been a powerful spiritual guide. Without her and her introduction to Martha Harrell and Randy Sherman, I am not sure how I would have made it through the challenges in my life. Shivaun, Martha, and Randy, your support and investment in my growth have enabled me to invest similarly in others' growth.

In my darkest and brightest times, I have often relied on the unconditional generosity, love, and support of my "Well Pack." Lisa, Bailey, EJ, Lara, Jennifer, Lynn, Edna, Nicole, and Susi: you have carried me on the path when I couldn't walk alone. With you, my spirit is continually replenished.

For forty-seven years my parents, Karen and Perry Jaster, have been my biggest cheerleaders. From reading me *Free to Be You and Me* to taking me to Science on Saturdays, showing me how to use imagination and ingenuity to make something from nothing and teaching me that you can do or be anything if you put your mind to it, they never missed a beat to be creative, thoughtful, and dedicated in their parenting. Their support and unconditional love are extraordinary.

Mom and Dad: *This* is my treehouse, so I will now let that go.

Writing a book is like climbing a mountain. It is an incredible challenge made infinitely better with a great team. Standing on the top of this mountain, I must shout the praises of my gifted writing partner, Val Frankel. This book would not exist without her. Her support, wisdom, and enthusiasm throughout this process were of immeasurable value. She manifested my vision so expertly and made it fun. She is a gift, my soul mate. Much gratitude goes to Alex Glass, literary agent extraordinaire who coached me through countless decisions with my best interests always at heart. With Alex and Val, I was part of an amazing team, and then there was Julie Will, my editor at Harper Wave, and the team became exceptional. Julie's incredible spirit, enthusiasm, and tireless edits made this book polished and succinct. Writing and editing a book are long, challenging processes filled with question marks and run-on sentences, and I am convinced that there would have been a lot more sleepless nights without her extraordinary commitment.

Last but not least, I must give credit to my wonderfully supportive husband, David Wannen, for embracing every zany adventure I have dreamed up. His commitment to our family is unwavering through every storm, and his love for us is endless and enduring.

Dave, you are proof that the Universe loves me, and I am blessed beyond words to hike through life with you.

OH HERE IS LOVE, AND HERE IS TRUTH.

—W. S. GILBERT

Index